Nurses'
Responses
to Patients'
Suffering

Lois Leiderman Davitz, Ph.D., received her bachelor's degree from The University of Michigan and master's and doctoral degrees from Columbia University. She has been associated with the department of nursing education at Teachers College, Columbia University since 1964. She was coprincipal investigator of the research project, Nurses' Inferences of Physical Pain and Psychological Distress. Author of *Interpersonal Processes in Nursing: Case Histories, The Psychiatric Patient: Case Histories,* and coauthor of several other books, Dr. Davitz has published many articles on research and nursing in professional journals. In addition to her work in the United States she has been lecturer and coordinator of nursing conferences and workshops in various parts of Africa.

Joel R. Davitz, Ph.D., received his bachelor's degree from the University of Illinois and his doctoral degree from Columbia University. Since 1955 he has been on the faculty of Teachers College, Columbia University and is currently Professor of Psychology and Education. Author of *Language of Emotion, The Communication of Emotional Meaning,* and coauthor of several other books, Dr. Davitz has published extensively in professional journals. He served as coprincipal investigator of the research project, Nurses' Inferences of Physical Pain and Psychological Distress. In addition, Dr. Davitz has served as consultant on a wide variety of nursing projects and as participant in nursing education workshops and conferences.

Charlene Fischi Rubin, B.S.N.E., M.A., Me.D., received her B.S.N.E. from Misericordia College and her master's degrees from Teachers College, Columbia University. She has been employed in a variety of administrative positions and for many years served as Associate Director of Nursing at St. Luke's Hospital. Ms. Rubin is completing her doctoral studies at Teachers College, Columbia University and is currently a member of the faculty of the nursing department. Her specialty area is quality assurance and she has published many articles in professional nursing journals.

Nurses' Responses to Patients' Suffering

Lois Leiderman Davitz
Joel Robert Davitz
with
Charlene Fischi Rubin

Springer Publishing Company   *New York*

Springer Publishing Company, Inc.
200 Park Avenue South
New York, New York 10003

80 81 82 83 84 / 10 9 8 7 6 5 4 3 2 1

Library of Congress Cataloging in Publication Data

Davitz, Lois Jean.
 Nurses' responses to patients' suffering.

 Bibliography: p.
 Includes index.
 1. Nursing—Psychological aspects. 2. Pain—Nursing
 3. Nurse and patient. 4. Suffering. I. Davitz, Joel
 Robert, joint author II. Rubin, Charlene Fischi,
 joint author. III. Title. [DNLM: 1. Nurse—Patient
 relations. 2. Nursing care—Psychology. 3. Attitude
 of health personnel. WY87 D265n]
 RT.86.D39   1980   610.73   80-13689
 ISBN 0-8261-2920-X
 ISBN 0-8261-2921-8 (pbk.)

Printed in the United States of America

Contents

Acknowledgments

We would like to express our profound appreciation to the many individuals who contributed so much to the successful completion of the various studies that lead us to write *Nurses' Responses to Patients' Suffering*. We wish to thank the directors of nursing of the forty-five cooperating hospitals. Their outstanding cooperation, invaluable suggestions, and continual support were extremely important to all phases of the investigation. We are deeply indebted to the eight thousand professional nurses in the United States who were actively involved in one or several of the studies. We also want to thank the fourteen hundred nurses from Japan, Korea, Thailand, Israel, Uganda, Belgium, Nigeria, England, Nepal, India, Puerto Rico, and Taiwan for their participation in the cross-cultural phases of the research. To these individuals, and to countless others who were involved in various stages of this research, we extend our respect and deep sense of gratitude.

This research was supported by Grant No. NU 00497 from the Nursing Research Branch, Division of Nursing, Department of Health, Education and Welfare.

LOIS LEIDERMAN DAVITZ, PH.D.
JOEL ROBERT DAVITZ, PH.D.
Research Assistants:
YASUKO HIGUCHI, B.S., R.N., ED.D.
ELIZABETH VECCHIONE, B.S., R.N., M.A.
GERALDINE VERRASSI, B.S., R.N., M.ED.

Introduction

Regardless of time, place, language, or culture, responding to patient suffering is a central aspect of nursing. Because coping with patient pain and psychological distress is a major part of professional nursing practice, understanding the process of how nurses judge patient suffering is extremely important.

For the past six years, under grants from the Division of Nursing of the Department of Health, Education and Welfare, we have been investigating factors that influence nurses' judgments about the degree of suffering experienced by patients. This volume is based on the results of the research. The goal of our research has been to identify and describe those factors that determine how nurses think about patients' pain and psychological distress, and to investigate the relation between nurses' beliefs about suffering and the way they interact with patients.

We began with the consideration that the suffering of another person is necessarily inferred rather than directly observed. No one can directly observe another person's experience. All we can do is observe behaviors. For example, assume that you have a headache. You point to your temples, tell us how much your head hurts, and describe the throbbing sensations you're experiencing. We can offer sympathy and medication, but no matter how sensitive or empathic we are, we cannot directly feel *your* headache. Our knowledge of your headache depends on what you say, how you look, and how you behave. We cannot experience your discomfort. All we can do is make a judgment or an inference about how you feel, and these judgments reflect our beliefs about your suffering.

Our judgment about your suffering depends upon your behavior and how we interpret that behavior. For example, while describing how awful your head felt, let's say you were smiling and making humorous comments. The fact that you were smiling and joking might prompt us to doubt that you were really feeling miserable. We might believe that someone who is suffering doesn't usually have a happy expression or make many jokes. We may, of course, be wrong. Perhaps you really were distressed, but you are the kind of person who covers up feelings; you handle pain by masking your real feelings with humor. Since we cannot feel your pain, however, we make a judgment about how much your head hurts, and that judgment depends on our belief system. In our opinion, a smile, laughter, and humorous comments typically indicate a feeling of well-being; therefore, despite your report of a headache, we judge your discomfort as relatively minor.

Every time you work with a patient, your beliefs about suffering influence the judgments you make about how much pain or psychological distress the patient is experiencing. And these judgments, in turn, determine how you behave in relation to that patient. If you believe that the patient is suffering a great deal, you may go out of your way to provide pain medication, sympathetic psychological support, and special nursing care. On the other hand, even if the patient complains a lot, if you don't think he is suffering very much, you may not be very sympathetic and, you may provide only routine care, without the extra time and effort you might devote to those patients whom you believe are "really" suffering.

Thus, nurses' beliefs about suffering make an enormous difference in their judgments about patients and in the ways they care for their patients. Our research, therefore, focused on these beliefs in an effort to understand more fully the process of nursing and to develop a research foundation for the continuing improvement of nursing care.

The studies summarized in this volume fall into several major categories. First, we were concerned with how certain characteristics of patients influenced nurses' judgments of suffering. Does a patient's age, for example, make a difference in the degree of physical pain or psychological distress a nurse might believe that patient is experiencing? Do nurses believe that young children and adults differ in the suffering they experience? Similarly, does a patient's socioeconomic class make a difference in nurses' judgments? Does the fact that a patient is rich or poor influence nurses' beliefs about the degree of pain or psychological distress that patient is feeling? Do other factors, such as a patient's sex or ethnic background, play a part in determining nurses' inferences of suffering? These are the kinds of questions we investigated in our first series of studies, and the results of this research and their implications for nursing are considered in the first section of this book.

We then turned out attention to nurses' beliefs about the degree of suffering associated with various illnesses and injuries. Obviously, the nature of a patient's illness or injury makes a difference in what the patient experiences. Some illnesses involve a great deal of pain; other illnesses are relatively painless. Some illnesses elicit a high degree of psychological distress; other illnesses may have very little psychological effect. Our major question was: What do nurses believe about the degree of suffering associated with various illnesses and injuries? What conditions are thought to be especially painful? Are these the same conditions that nurses view as psychologically very distressful? What is the relationship between nurses' beliefs about the level of pain involved in various illnesses and injuries and their beliefs about the degree of psychological distress associated with these conditions? In general, do nurses believe that patients typically experience relatively greater pain or greater psychological distress? The answers to these questions provide important insights into the system of beliefs that many nurses share and thus contribute a great deal to our understanding of the nursing process.

Throughout the early stages of our research, we noticed that, while nurses shared certain beliefs about suffering, they also had many individual differences. Although our research showed that nurses agreed, for example, that some illnesses were typically more painful or psychologically more distressful than other illnesses, there were consistent differences among nurses in their assessments of the overall level of pain of the particular patient or the particular illness considered; some nurses believed that the patient suffered relatively little, while other nurses believed that the same patient suffered a great deal. This observation led us to our investigations of individual and cultural differences among nurses. First, we established the fact that nurses consistently differ in the overall level of suffering they infer about patients. Then, we investigated a number of variables that might account for these individual differences. Do the nurses' different areas of specialization make a difference in the degree of suffering they infer? Are years of nursing experience related to judgments about suffering? Do the nurses' own experiences with pain influence the degree of pain they infer in patients? Do the ethnic backgrounds of nurses make a difference? These are only a few of the questions considered in this section.

We expanded this aspect of our research by studying nurses in a number of different countries. Through the cooperation of nurses in many different parts of the world, we were able to compare judgments of patients' suffering made by nurses in Japan, Korea, Uganda, Israel, and a number of other countries. As a result of this research, we have a greater understanding of how cultural differences are reflected in nurses' beliefs, and on the basis of these cross-cultural comparisons, perhaps we can gain greater awareness of our own attitudes and beliefs.

Athough the studies of nurses' beliefs are interesting and worthwhile in and of themselves, a very significant part of our research related nurses' beliefs about suffering to the ways in which they behaved with patients. Common sense suggests that beliefs should be meaningfully related to behavior, but sometimes this does not turn out to be true. We therefore designed our research to test the general hypothesis that nurses' beliefs are related to their behaviors, and to determine more specifically the ways in which beliefs about suffering are reflected in particular nursing actions. In our initial research along this line, we studied nurses in medical-surgical units interacting with their patients. The results of this research were very promising, but in the course of this research, it occurred to us that the situation in which a nurse worked may influence the relationship between her beliefs and her behaviors. In medical-surgical units, we found a clear and consistent relation between nurses' beliefs about suffering and certain nursing behaviors, but we did not know whether this same pattern would hold true in other nursing situations. To investigate this issue, therefore, we repeated our research in two other, quite different settings: in pediatric units and in obstetric units. Both of these settings differ in many respects from the typical medical-surgical setting, and thus provided a basis for comparing the ways in which beliefs and behaviors are related in different kinds of nursing situations.

As part of our overall research project, we talked to a large number of nurses about their reactions to patients' suffering. These interviews provided many important insights and leads for further research. One of the most interesting concerned the differences between nurses' reactions in their current practice and their reactions when they began nursing training. This led us to study the changes in nursing students' beliefs about patients' suffering over the course of their nursing education. The results of this research showed some very clear-cut patterns of change during nursing education, but the finding that will perhaps prove to be most interesting to nursing educators as well as to practicing nurses is the difference between changing beliefs about pain and changing beliefs about psychological distress. Both of these sets of beliefs change significantly during a nurse's education, but they change in opposite directions. This finding will be discussed in greater detail in Chapter 10, where we will also consider some of the implications of these results.

In Chapter 12 of this volume, we asked Charlene Rubin, who has had a wide range of experience in nursing and nursing administration, to discuss the results of our research from the perspective of a nurse administrator. This discussion is an extremely valuable supplement to our investigations, providing a very useful bridge between theory and research, on the one hand, and the everyday realities of nursing practice, on the other.

1

The Effects of
a Patient's Social Class
on Nurses' Inferences of Suffering

Janice Lowry, a 37-year-old woman, a well known fashion designer, flew to Switzerland for a ski holiday. The intensive pressures of her work were such that getting away for a vacation was absolutely necessary before she was caught up in the frenetic pace of Christmas activities. The second day of the trip, while trying out a new pair of skis, she fell and fractured her right arm. The unfortunate accident not only ruined her plans, but interrupted her social and work commitments. "With an arm in a cast," she commented, "there's not much one can really wear or /do. It's awful any time, but even worse now with all that's on my calendar. I don't know how I'm going to manage."

Clarice Tipton, 35 years of age, has been employed as a night cleaning woman in a large office building. "I like working at night," she told her supervisor. "I got time to spend with my five kids. I can't let them run the streets. This way I'm home for lunch and after school. I sleep in between."

While waxing the corridors one evening, she stumbled and struck her right arm on the metal edge of a water cooler. Her arm was fractured. Workman's Compensation didn't cover her living costs. "I need my job. I don't want welfare. I've never been on welfare. It would hurt my pride. I got five kids and I manage." Without the use of her right arm, she was overwhelmed. "I can't even get my housework done. It had to happen right before the holidays. It's got me down." Divorced, Ms. Tipton is the sole support of her family.

We discussed these two cases with a group of nurses. Both patients were about the same age and had similar injuries. Did they suffer the same or different amounts of physical pain and psychological distress as a consequence of their fractured arms?

"It's a lot worse for Ms. Tipton," one nurse told us.

"What do you mean by worse?" we asked.

"It's bound to mean more to her. She has a family. The children to take care of—herself. She needs that job. I don't know how she works nights and runs a house. It must be awful for her now with her arm in a cast."

"And Ms. Lowry?" we added.

"A fractured arm on a ski trip in Switzerland? My heart isn't bleeding for her."

"Do you think her arm hurts as much? The report shows that the fractures are just about the same."

"I don't think so. She'll survive."

"How about their psychological distress?"

"I can't even compare the two women," we were told. "A night cleaning woman and a fashion designer in Switzerland for a holiday? Ms. Tipton probably doesn't spend in a month what that trip cost Ms. Lowry."

Whether one judges there to be more or less pain as the result of an accident while skiing or an accident while working at night mopping floors is an individual matter. There isn't a right or wrong answer to the questions we raised. Any answer is a personal judgment or a belief.

While we sat in the nurses' lounge talking with the staff during a coffee break, one nurse told us about a patient who had been admitted to the unit the previous evening. He was 50 years of age and had had a myocardial infarction.

"I really feel for the man."

"Why?"

"The pressure he's under. He's president of the bank here in town. He's driven himself. He recognizes this now, but it's too late. His wife and kids were here. He's quite a VIP. You should have seen the way people were hopping around taking care of him. It's going to take time, but he'll pull through."

Later that afternoon, we were in the emergency room. Two attendants brought in a patient on a stretcher. The man appeared to be in his 60s; however, identification papers showed that he was 49. There was no money in his wallet, or papers showing employment or place of residence. The name of a woman, his sister, was pinned to an inner pocket of his coat. The diagnosis was myocardial infarction.

The nurses attended to his needs quickly and efficiently. After they had completed their tasks, we talked to them.

"Is he suffering a great deal of pain?"

"He's not in pain now. But it was rough on him for awhile," one of the staff told us. "He's lucky someone called the police."

"How about his psychological distress? How do you think he's going to feel about all of this?"

"Bad, like anyone. But he's been through hell. All of us were surprised to find out that he wasn't as old as we thought at first. This probably is nothing compared to some things that must have happened to him, judging by the way he looks."

In many respects, these two patients shared much in common. Both were males about the same age and had the identical diagnosis. The principal difference between them was their social class background. Does the fact that one patient is poor and another wealthy make a difference in the way nurses judge physical pain and psychological distress? Reactions to sufferings of other people are likely to differ among any group of people. For some, perhaps, an accident to Ms. Tipton, a hardworking woman with a modest income and a family to support, is far worse than an injury to an individual like Ms. Lowry, who is wealthy and successful. In other instances, some people might judge the bank president's illness as far more debilitating than the same illness to an individual who has far less responsibility to the community or to a family. The feeling might be that the unemployed man who has suffered a great deal is more accustomed to physical discomfort.

Reasonable people with similar backgrounds may differ greatly in their judgments about the extent of pain or distress another person suffers. We may all be convinced of the rightness of our own judgments, certain that those with opposite opinions are completely mistaken. No matter how confident we might feel about our own opinions, however, the fact remains that people's opinions do differ.

Many factors influence the judgments nurses make about patients. One of these variables is social class, and the research problem we investigated was designed to answer the question of whether nurses' inferences of suffering were related to a patient's socioeconomic background. Does it make a difference in the nurses' judgments if a patient is from a low-, middle-, or upper-class background? From the nurses' perspectives, would the suffering of people differ if, in all respects other than social class, these patients are very much alike?

Nurses who participated in the study ranged in age and nursing experience. The sample included nurses from a variety of socioeconomic backgrounds. All were employed in a variety of specialty areas in hospital settings at the time the study was made.

The nurses were presented with a series of brief descriptions of patients and asked to rate the degree of physical pain and the degree of psychological distress they felt the patients were likely to be experiencing. The items included information about the age, sex, nature of illness or injury, and social class of a patient. Three social classes were identified: low, middle, and high. The classification of occupations into social classes was based on a standard scale developed as a sociological tool. Lower-class occupations included, for example, janitors, maids, and waitresses. Middle-class occupations included newspaper reporters, editors, lab technicians, policemen, and so forth. Upper-class occupations included, for example, physicians, newspaper editors, and business executives.

The following examples show how the information was presented for a given illness, social class, and sex category. In all three instances, the patients were male and had low-grade systolic murmurs. The difference was in the social class. One patient was president of a large consulting firm, another was a janitor, and the third patient a master electrician. Although the three items are presented together in the illustration, the order of the items in the final questionnaire, for all illnesses, classes, and both sexes, was *random*.

Kurt Oates, president of a large consulting firm, was feeling the effects of business pressures and thought he should have a physical checkup. A low-grade systolic murmur was discovered, and further diagnostic tests were ordered.

Physical Pain, Discomfort:	1	2	3	4	5	6	7
Psychological Distress:	1	2	3	4	5	6	7

Leonard Benson, 38 years of age, was hospitalized for diagnostic studies as a result of routine physical examination required by the civil service prior to his being appointed as a janitor. A low-grade systolic murmur was noted.

Physical Pain, Discomfort:	1	2	3	4	5	6	7
Psychological Distress:	1	2	3	4	5	6	7

Diagnosed as having a low-grade systolic murmur, Harry Graves, 36 years of age, was admitted to the hospital. A self-employed master electrician, he was advised by his doctor to undergo a complete series of tests.

Physical Pain, Discomfort:	1	2	3	4	5	6	7
Psychological Distress:	1	2	3	4	5	6	7

The task for the nurses was to read each item and, on the basis of their judgments, rate the degree of physical pain and the degree of psychological distress they felt the patient was experiencing. We were interested in the nurses' opinions, their judgments about each patient's situation. This was not a test. There were no right or wrong answers. We were only interested in nurses' judgments.

In the various questionnaires, we included illnesses and injuries from the following areas: cardiovascular, trauma, psychiatric, cancer, and infection. For every illness or injury, there were six items. Three of the items concerned male patients from each social class, and three concerned female patients from each social class.

This procedure of having separate items for each different illness or injury, and for different ages, sex, and social classes, was followed throughout all the questionnaires. Our overall goal was to study the relationship between patients' social class backgrounds and nurses' inferences of suffering. Thus, all the information, with the exception of social class, was relatively the same for a particular illness or injury, male or female patients, and age group.

Findings

The results were striking. The social class of the patient did make a difference in the degree of physical pain and psychological distress nurses felt patients experienced. We must keep clearly in mind that we were only concerned with nurses' judgments about the suffering of others and *not* how much suffering the patients may have felt they actually experienced.

According to nurses, lower-class patients, both male and female, were judged to suffer more pain with the same illness or injury than were middle- or upper-class patients. One nurse commented to us when we reported the findings at one session, "It hurts more when you're poor. A woman like Ms. Tipton has more on her mind, more to worry about." This, of course, is the nurse's judgment. Perhaps if we had talked to a woman like Ms. Lowry, her reactions to pain might have been that no one had suffered as much as she was suffering at that moment. It is very much a matter of one's perspective.

The sex of the patient also made a difference when considered in conjunction with social class. That is, when judgments about the suffering of lower-class females were compared to judgments about lower-class males, the females were viewed as suffering greater physical pain than males. The opposite was true for upper-class patients. That is, an upper-class man who had a myocardial infarction, for example, and was about 50 years of age, was judged to suffer more than an upper-class woman who was the same age, with the same diagnosis. In discussing their reactions to upper-class males and females, the nurses reasoned that for a man, it is much harder to be inactive during the recovery period, or that the man is the main financial support in the family. Another response was that, "In my experience, the more successful a man is, the worse he seems to react to pain." Again, these are judgments made by nurses about the pain of others and may, indeed, be quite different from the pain actually experienced by the patients.

Judgments about psychological distress in patients were also influenced by the socioeconomic backgrounds of the individual patients. For example, nurses believed that lower-class patients suffered greater psychological distress with certain illnesses than did upper- or middle-class patients. In particular, lower-class patients who had myocardial infarctions, for example, were believed to have far less psychological distress than middle- or upper-class patients.

The sex of a patient made considerable difference in the judgments made about patient distress. Middle-class female patients, for example, were assumed to suffer much less distress than middle-class male patients, although they all had relatively the same age and injury or illness.

The specific way nurses judged patients from different socioeconomic backgrounds is intriguing, of course. However, the really important conclusion of the study is that the social class of patients makes a significant difference in nurses' judgments about how much pain and psychological distress patients experience.

All of us have certain beliefs that influence the ways in which we see our world and interpret what goes on around us. To a certain extent, these beliefs are based on evidence we have obtained, either from our own direct experiences or from the experiences of others, although we also have some beliefs that are based on very little evidence. We may react in one way to a bank president and in a quite different way to an unemployed laborer, partly as a result of our beliefs about people from different socioeconomic classes. But for the most part, these beliefs may not make a great deal of practical difference in our lives or in the lives of others. We generally accept the fact that people have different beliefs, and we usually learn to live with these differences.

For nursing, however, these beliefs can make an enormous difference in the care given to patients. If a nurse believes that a cleaning woman with a broken arm suffers more pain than a wealthy fashion designer with exactly the same injury, it is more than likely that the nurse will pay particular attention to the cleaning woman's pain and perhaps even discount the pain of the woman who is a fashion designer. Yet, both women are patients. Each experiences some degree of pain, and each deserves the nurse's individual attention and professional care, regardless of the difference in socioeconomic status.

Similarly, the bank president and the laborer with a myocardial infarction may both be experiencing psychological distress that has little or nothing to do with how much money each has, how big or small a house they live in, or what part of town they come from. Each may feel threatened by the illness in his own way, and each should receive the nursing care that he needs. If nurses believe that wealthier people suffer more psychological distress than do poorer people, they may well emphasize psychological aspects of care with the wealthier patients and perhaps neglect this aspect of nursing care with the poorer patients.

Thus, in their professional role, nurses cannot permit the beliefs, biases, and stereotypes that operate in everyday life to influence their nursing care. Every patient is an individual who experiences his or her own unique pain and unique psychological distress, and effective nursing must be based on a recognition of each patient's individuality.

The findings of our research, therefore, suggest that individual nurses should examine their personal beliefs about patients from different social classes. As a result of this self-examination, a nurse may become aware of these personal beliefs and biases, and thus be able to guard against stereotypes that sometimes interfere with providing the nursing care that is best for each individual patient.

2

The Effects of a Patient's Age on Nurses' Inferences of Suffering

The patient, a 22-year-old male, was admitted to the hospital for a series of tests to determine whether or not the young man had cancer. Several days later, the diagnosis was confirmed, and a program of treatment was scheduled. The prognosis for recovery was poor.

The entire nursing staff was extremely upset. "Hearing this kind of diagnosis about any patient on the floor always leaves everyone with an empty feeling," commented one nurse. "You have to face the fact that there's nothing you can do to change the inevitable way the case is going to end, and that's what makes it hard."

Several of the nurses found it impossible to work with the young man. One stated, "I have to push myself to go into the room. To have his life end before he really had a chance to live is very disturbing to me. I'm so afraid he'll 'read' the expression on my face. This always happens to me when a young person comes into the hospital and I know they're not going to walk out of here recovered."

Two of the staff, who had been in practice less than a year, recalled breaking down when they heard the news. One reported, "My friend and I went into the lounge and started to cry. We couldn't stop. We'd look at each other and know what we were thinking and we'd break into tears. I know we kept thinking we're the same age as that guy. How could we ever take knowing this about ourselves. We felt like we were walking around in a daze all that week."

In a room at the end of the same corridor, an 87-year-old man had a similar diagnosis. Both he and his family knew that it was only a matter of weeks before he died. The patient was alert, and relatively comfortable, despite his increasing weakness. Although the staff felt saddened to see his deteriorating condition, the reactions were quite different from their attitude toward the 22-year-old. "When I go in to see this elderly man," said one nurse, "I'm not depressed. I'm sorry for him and do what I can, but it isn't an unhappy experience. He's gentle and sweet. Yesterday, he told me he has lived a long, full life and he's not afraid to die. He even said to me that it's harder for his children and grandchildren than it is for him. I came away from the room feeling stronger myself about death, which has always bothered me. Talking to him is very inspiring."

Both patients were male, and both were dying. The one significant difference between the two men was their age. On the basis of discussions with nurses and observations of their reactions to people of varying ages, it seemed reasonable to raise the question of whether a patient's age made a difference in nurses' judgments about suffering.

In order to study the effects of a patient's age on nurses' judgments, therefore, we developed a series of questionnaires that included descriptions of patients with various illnesses in four age brackets: young children between the ages of 4 and 12; late adolescents and young adults between the ages of 17 and 25; older adults between the ages of 30 and 45; elderly individuals over 65. Both male and female patients were included in each age group.

Nurses who volunteered to respond to the questionnaires ranged in age. All had been professionally employed in a variety of hospital settings from a minimum of several years to a maximum of more than twenty.

Findings

The age of the patient appeared to have little influence on nurses' inferences of physical pain. For example, one series of items was about patients who had to undergo surgery for repair of an aortic aneurysm. In general, the nurses judged the degree of pain associated with this condition to be the same regardless of the age or sex of the patient. According to the ratings, a young boy or girl would have about the same pain as a young male or female adolescent, a middle-aged man or woman, or an elderly man or woman.

Although nurses' judgments about physical pain were not influenced by the age of the patient, age did play an important role in nurses' inferences of psychological distress. Nurses believed that children, ages 4 to 12, experienced considerably less psychological distress than any older age group.

"Children do not really understand the meaning of their illnesses," one nurse commented. Other nurses with whom we discussed these findings agreed with the interpretation. There are exceptions; however, in general, the nurses felt that young, hospitalized children were unable to fully understand the implications of their illnesses or injuries. "I've worked on both pediatric units and adult 'med-surgical' units," said one nurse. "And I've been amazed at the difference. Take a child with thrombophlebitis, one of the illnesses on the questionnaire. The child will want to get going, can't see any reason to have to stay in bed. The child isn't at all concerned about the implications of the condition. It doesn't help to use scare tactics to get the child to stay quiet. With adults, they'll want to know what the condition means. When the doctor explains some of the implications, they may get frightened or worried."

Other nurses with whom we discussed this finding agreed that young children cannot always understand the meaning of their illnesses or conditions and are, therefore, less likely to be psychologically upset. One nurse gave the following report of a personal experience. As a child, the nurse had fractured a radial bone while sledding. After the initial pain had subsided, the condition was "fun." The child was the center of attention at home, and the arm in a cast covered with autographs was a sensation among the child's friends. "I didn't stop anything at school, even gym. As a child, it doesn't matter. But I remember a patient I had, a man in his 40s, who had the same kind of fracture I had as a kid. He became so depressed when his arm was put in a cast. I can understand. He was a carpenter; this accident meant he couldn't work. The implications of the injury had real meaning for him. It wasn't a lark.''

The results of our study show that nurses, in general, believe that when children are ill or injured, they suffer less psychological distress than adults with equivalent illnesses or injuries suffer. And our discussions with nurses suggest that this judgment is based on their assumption that children do not understand as fully as do adults the consequences and possible implications of their physical condition.

This finding and the reasoning underlying nurses' judgments about children clearly reflect an adult's point of view. For an adult, the psychological distress associated with illness may be based largely on concerns about what will happen as a result of the illness. The person's life may be more or less seriously disrupted; there may be some long-term disability involved; financial worries may add to the stress; and in some conditions, the possibility of death may be a source of anxiety. All of this, of course, requires some degree of understanding. Thus, from an adult's perspective, one might reason that, if children understand less about the implications and possible consequences of their conditions, they are less likely to worry about what might happen. In this sense, then, children's lack of knowledge and understanding may protect them from psychological distress.

Although this reasoning undoubtedly has some validity, it neglects the very important possibility that the major source of a child's anxiety may be somewhat different from that of adults. Separation from parents and the unfamiliar environment of the hospital can be extremely threatening to a child and give rise to intense fear. The lack of understanding itself, the possible misunderstanding of what is happening, the pain, and for the child, the mysterious events sometimes encountered during hospitalization, can make the child extremely anxious.

In our observations and discussions with pediatric nurses, it is clear that the great majority of nurses who work primarily with children are well aware of these possible sources of psychological distress among children. On the basis of their experience, they recognize that ill or injured children can very well be as anxious as any adult patient, and effective pediatric care depends, in part, on sensitivity to this distress. Our study, however, indicates that other nurses, those who work largely with adults, may not empathize as fully as they might with children. As a result, there may be some tendency to discount the degree of psychological distress experienced by young patients. It would therefore be important to recognize that the causes of fear, anxiety, and worry for adults and children may sometimes differ, but both children and adults may suffer equivalent degrees of psychological distress, regardless of differences in age.

3

The Effects of a Patient's Ethnic, National, and Religious Background on Nurses' Inferences of Suffering

Marie Sanchez, 26 years of age, insisted that her husband take her directly to the hospital the minute she felt her first labor pain. The doctor had told her to wait until the pains came on a regular basis, but at the onset of labor, Ms. Sanchez began weeping and rushed to the hospital. During the admissions process, she clung to her husband, providing only mumbled, tearful responses to questions.

"I'm worried about my wife," Mr. Sanchez told the nurse. "Please get the doctor. I called him. Please, you call. Tell him to come. It's an emergency."

"It's not an emergency," the nurse answered him. "Millions of women go through this without any trouble. Your wife is just fine."

Later, when Ms. Sanchez was helped into bed, still weeping, the nurse told her, "You're not doing yourself or the baby any good by carrying on like this."

Ms. Sanchez was in labor for ten hours. During that time, she never ceased to express her discomfort, sobbing, and crying. The nurses who attended her could do very little to get her to calm down and relax. Her response to any of these requests was to increase the volume of her sobs. A healthy, eight-pound boy was born shortly after midnight. The entire delivery had been routine, and Ms. Sanchez, after a first admiring look at her son, slept soundly the rest of the night.

One of the nurses voiced irritation with Ms. Sanchez. "There was absolutely no need for her to act like she did. I could understand if she had something wrong. That wasn't the case. She was perfectly healthy. Of course, there is pain, but she only made it worse."

Was Ms. Sanchez "putting on a good show," as this nurse thought? Were the patient's cries forced and purposeful? Obviously, the nurse could not believe Ms. Sanchez was suffering to any great degree.

We talked to Ms. Sanchez the following day about her experience. Had she been in extreme pain? Why had she cried? At first, Ms. Sanchez was puzzled by the questions. According to her, she had expressed her feelings. "Puerto Rican people," she told us, "are expressive. When we are happy, we laugh. When we are upset, we cry. All my friends told me how much they cried during labor. I never believed them. Now I do. My grandmother always told me, 'You cry hard when the baby is born and you have a healthy baby.' I am glad it is over. I feel fine."

For Ms. Sanchez, childbirth was associated with pain, and her cries and complaints were natural. Ms. Sanchez was extremely vocal during labor. According to some nurses, other Puerto Rican women tended to react similarly. "It's not like that in my country," a Nigerian nurse told us.

We had the opportunity to observe Nigerian women at a maternity clinic in Lagos. About seventy women waited in a lounge to be admitted to the clinic. All were expecting their babies within the next several hours. There wasn't an audible sound in the room. Each of the women was taken in turn to the delivery floor where she was examined and prepped for the delivery. Rarely did a woman express discomfort during the examination and the delivery. There were no tears, no shouts, no complaints. From our observations, the women appeared to be relaxed. The deliveries proceeded without complications, and seldom did any of them require anesthetic or medication to alleviate pain. With the exception of a few women, the majority remained in the hospital for less than twenty-four hours. Several had walked away unassisted from the delivery room to their beds where they rested for a short period of time.

We asked several women how much pain they had experienced.

Had they felt like shouting or crying? One woman smiled at our query. She told us that her mother had had ten children, which she delivered by herself. "She went out to the fields, had the baby, and carried it home to the family. She was very proud of being able to do this. I told her women go to the hospitals or clinics today. It was not true for my mother or her friends."

"Did you feel like doing anything or asking for medicine when the pain was bad?" we asked another patient.

"Why?" was the response. "The pain was not bad enough for medicine. I knew it would all be over in a little while."

In the first example, the nurse had a difficult time accepting Ms. Sanchez's expressions of agony during what the nurse felt was a normal process of labor and delivery. For this nurse and others, Puerto Rican women tended to over-dramatize their discomfort. In the second example, we had difficulty accepting the patients' equanimity and reserve. We automatically assumed that Nigerian women, who in other situations impressed us as being outgoing and expressive, would behave in a similar way during childbirth.

To what extent do our beliefs or expectations about different groups affect our judgments and behaviors? In one case, a Jewish man who had been recently hospitalized was lying quietly in bed, reading. The nurse entered the room and began talking with him. "There's no need to get all upset. You'll be fine. I know you're in pain. You don't have to keep asking for medication. We'll take care of you."

He told us that he had not put on his call light, and had not complained or requested medication. "Every time one of the nurses came in to see me, I had this feeling they were expecting me to complain. I wanted to ask them what it was all about."

We talked with the nurses about their reactions to this 45-year-old Jewish man. One nurse told us that, in her experience, Jewish men seem to hurt a lot worse than other patients. Because this Jewish man did not complain or make requests, the nurses' repeated implications that he was demanding were confusing for him. He wondered what was going on in the nurses' minds. Was there something far worse wrong with him than he realized?

This raises the question of what happens when a patient from a particular group *doesn't* conform to the stereotypes we may have about that culture. In one instance, we observed a middle-aged Oriental man who came into the emergency room of a large metropolitan hospital. He had broken his arm, and he sobbed uncontrollably. The head nurse told us that the staff members were momentarily taken aback. "We've had lots of Oriental patients and they've always been stoic. Not a sound. The nurses were stunned. They had never had an Oriental patient react in such an extreme way."

One of the nurses who had been jarred by the situation said that her first thought had been, "What is an Oriental man doing crying?" She told us that she had felt uncomfortable thinking this way, but it was the first thought that flashed through her mind.

As a result of these kinds of observations, we decided to study nurses' attitudes toward different ethnic, national, and religious groups. The general question we raised was: Are nurses' inferences of suffering related to the ethnic, national, or religious background of their patients? That is, do nurses as a group share a particular set of beliefs about patients from various backgrounds? Does a nurse, for example, have certain expectations about the degree of suffering a Jewish person experiences? An Oriental, Mediterranean, Black, Spanish, Anglo-Saxon, or German? Does the nature of the illness, together with the ethnic background, affect the nurses' judgments?

The nurses who participated in this study came from a variety of ethnic backgrounds. Ranging in age and experience, all were employed as staff or head nurses in a number of large metropolitan hospitals at the time of the study.

The questionnaire used in this study consisted of descriptions of male and female patients with various illnesses or injuries from the following ethnic or racial groups: Oriental, Mediterranean, Black, Spanish, Anglo-Saxon and Germanic, and Jewish. The following items are a few examples of *one* set of items that were randomly distributed throughout the questionnaire. In this case, the specific illness is psychiatric in origin. The patients were all female, between the ages of 26 and 37. Note that the one major difference among all five of these patients was their ethnic background. The rest of the descriptions are essentially the same.

Name: Juanita Delgado
Age: 29
Background: Puerto Rican
Symptoms: Nervous tension and irritability
Juanita Delgado went to her doctor seeking medication to calm her nerves. According to her report, lately she had been having "one bad day after another." Everything was upsetting her and "life seemed to be in a knot."

Name: Rita Foung
Age: 26
Background: Chinese
Symptoms: Nervousness and irritability
Rita Foung sought advice from a doctor. According to her statements, she had recently begun feeling "high-strung." She tended to overreact and was extremely sensitive about practically everything, which she felt was not her usual form of behavior.

Name: Alicia Columbo
Age: 29
Background: Italian
Symptoms: Irritability and tension
Friends suggested that Alicia Columbo go to the doctor for medication and advice. Recently she had become "cranky" and very nervous, "overreacting to everything."

Name: Cora Howard
Age: 34
Background: Black
Symptoms: Tension and nervousness
Cora Howard told the nurse that she had come to the doctor for

advice. Recently she had been bothered by her own nervous irritability, which didn't seem to wane. She didn't feel like herself because of this increasing nervous tension.

Name: Mary O'Hara
Age: 34
Background: Irish
Symptoms: Tension and nervousness

According to Mary O'Hara, she had always been a relatively easygoing person. Recently, she reported, she had found herself getting upset over minor occurrences and becoming moody and irritable about everyday matters that had never before troubled her.

Name: Sara Ginsburg
Age: 37
Background: Jewish
Symptoms: Nervous tension and irritability

Because of increasing irritability over minor events and a feeling that she was continually "ready to fly off the handle," Sara Ginsburg made an appointment to see a doctor. According to her, she was upset about small things and felt very edgy and sensitive.

Name: Anne McLaren
Age: 34
Background: Scottish
Symptoms: High anxiety and concern about the future

Anne McLaren sought help when she found herself feeling continually upset. "It's not my way or my family's way to be so anxious about every little thing." In addition, she felt that she saw the world in a new way, "as if everything is extremely sharp and defined." What was most upsetting was her extreme tension about the future.

Another set of items included descriptions of male patients with a specific illness or injury and from each of the same six ethnic backgrounds. An Anglo-Saxon patient might be designated as Irish, English, or Scottish; an Oriental patient might be Chinese, Japanese, and so forth; a Spanish patient might be Mexican, Puerto Rican, and so forth. Below each of the patient descriptions were two scales, one for physical pain and one for psychological distress. The nurses were asked to rate the patients on the degree of physical pain and psychological distress they felt each patient experienced. As with all the studies, we wanted the nurses' opinions. Our interest was *not* in how much suffering the patient felt he was experiencing, but rather the degree of suffering the nurses *believed* the patient experienced.

Findings

The results of the study showed that nurses infer different degrees of suffering for patients from various ethnic backgrounds. For example, the nurses who participated in the study very clearly judged Oriental and Anglo-Saxon or Germanic patients as having far less physical pain than Jewish or Spanish patients with identical conditions. Anglo-Saxon or Germanic patients, in particular, suffered minimal pain when they had a psychiatric illness. Oriental patients were judged to have minimal pain for trauma and cardiovascular diseases. The Jewish patient, regardless of the illness or injury, was judged by the nurses as suffering the greatest amount of pain. When the Jewish patient had a psychiatric illness or cardiovascular condition, the ratings for physical pain were extremely high.

Nurses' judgments for psychological distress closely paralleled their ratings for physical pain. Again, Oriental and Anglo-Saxon or Germanic patients were believed to suffer far less psychological distress with a given illness or condition than were Spanish or Jewish patients.

Thus, according to the nurses, Oriental and Anglo-Saxon or Germanic patients have the least pain and psychological distress; Jewish and Spanish patients experience the greatest suffering; and black and Mediterranean patients were rated in the middle, between the other groups.

The results of this study clearly show that the ethnic backgrounds of the patients influenced the nurses' judgments about suffering. Six patients, each from a different ethnic background, with identical illnesses or injuries, were judged differently. The one factor—ethnic background—made a significant difference in the ratings.

We may reasonably ask, to what extent do preconceived attitudes about a specific ethnic group affect our behavior? Appreciating the particular characteristics of a given ethnic group certainly may be helpful. For example, one nurse stated, "Knowing Puerto Rican patients react a lot helps me. I expect them to make their complaints known. I try to stay one step ahead of them. I never have any problems, because I am there first."

On the other hand, there may be times when the nurses' judgments may hinder nurse-patient relationships, particularly in those situations where the patient does not conform to the stereotypes. The Jewish man we spoke to had the feeling that the nurses expected him to complain. He felt they reacted to him as if he were demanding. In this instance, the nurses' belief system interfered with the development of a helpful nurse-patient relationship.

The problem for nursing is not simply a matter of doing away with all of our stereotypes. On the basis of previous research by Zborowski, we know that patients from various ethnic groups tend to react differently to the kinds of stress encountered when they are ill or injured.[1] Oriental patients, for example, tend to react more stoically than do Puerto Rican patients. In itself, this difference is neither good nor bad; it is a reflection of the different kinds of behavior expected of people in the two cultures. In general, a more stoic attitude towards pain is viewed as desirable in many Oriental cultures, while in the Puerto Rican culture, a person is expected to be more emotionally expressive.

Being aware of these cultural differences can be helpful to nurses who can learn to understand the behavior of patients in terms of their particular cultural backgrounds. Thus, nurses who are aware of cultural differences and understand patients in terms of their cultural backgrounds will respond more appropriately and effectively to the patients' needs. They will not be disturbed by the emotional ex-

---

[1]M. Zborowski, *People in Pain* (California: Jossey Bass, 1969).

pressiveness of a patient whose culture expects and encourages people to be very expressive, and will not mistake a more stoic attitude among patients from a different culture for a lack of feelings.

Nevertheless, any generalization about a cultural or ethnic group of people can blind us to differences among individuals within that group. It may be true that Chinese patients as a group are more stoic than Puerto Rican patients as a group. But within any group, there are enormous individual differences that must be recognized and appreciated by the nurse. In providing effective nursing care, the pain, the psychological distress, and the needs of the *individual* patient must be taken into account. Thus, even though there may be certain similarities among members of a particular ethnic group, nurses must be especially careful not to permit a stereotyped belief to interfere with their sensitivity to the individual patient.

Our research findings indicate that nurses do share more or less common beliefs about the suffering experienced by patients from different ethnic, national, and religious backgrounds. These beliefs may be based on common experiences with patients from these various groups, or they may stem from the stereotypes people share in the larger American culture. But regardless of the basis of these beliefs, in providing health care, nurses must be sensitive to the individuals who are their patients. Therefore, an important step in gaining this sensitivity to individuals is becoming aware of one's own generalized beliefs. If nurses are aware of their own beliefs about groups of people, they can guard against letting these generalizations distort their judgments about *individuals*. Through this kind of self-awareness and self-knowledge, nurses can achieve the awareness and understanding of others that is crucial in providing effective nursing care.

4
Nurses' Judgments of Pain and Distress Associated with Different Illnesses and Injuries

Ms. Rena, 47 years of age, entered the hospital for elective cosmetic surgery. She was scheduled to have bags underneath her eyes removed, her chin line tightened, and wrinkles from her forehead treated. During the postoperative period, she was very uncomfortable. She told nurses how much the operation hurt.

"The drawing sensation is terrible. I hate taking something to make me sleep, but I think I have to ask for some Demerol—or anything. Right here, at the side of my ears, it feels like someone has put pliers to my skin and is pulling. I never realized how miserable I was going to feel. The only thing that keeps me going is telling myself in another month I'll be myself—or almost myself. I can't wait to see how I look."

In another room at the opposite end of the corridor, Ms. Kent, 49 years old, grimaced and fitfully moaned at the slightest touch of a nurse's hands. As a result of a gas heater explosion, she had second-degree burns over her lower extremities. Despite all the nurses' care, Ms. Kent told the staff that she was in pain and begged for some medication to relieve the discomfort.

"I feel like my skin is being ripped from me, piece by piece. I never could imagine the pain I'm having. It's the worst I've ever felt. I suppose there'll come a day when I'll look back and not even remember what I felt like at this time."

From the point of view of each of these women, the pain was extremely hard to tolerate. Ms. Rena said the stitching on her face made her feel as if someone were tugging at her skin with pliers. Ms. Kent had similar sensations. She talked about feeling as if her skin were being torn from her limbs. Although the conditions resulted in pain and suffering for both women, from the point of view of the attending nurses, was the suffering experienced by Ms. Rena significantly different from the suffering experienced by Ms. Kent? We talked to a group of nurses about the two cases. The nurses were sympathetic; however, there were differences in their opinions about the degree of suffering they felt the patients experienced. One nurse commented, "Facial surgery does hurt. I know she's in pain, but she keeps calling for pills every hour. I told her she should try and hold out; we can't give her something for the pain every time she feels a twitch. She'll have to bear some discomfort. After all, no one made her redo her face. She had everything in one fell swoop. I do think she's exaggerating her pain. She wants attention."

She admitted that she felt far more compassion for Ms. Kent. "Everyone knows that burns can cause horrible pain. She has such an ordeal ahead of her. Skin grafts—I know it must be really difficult for her. There's only so much that we can do now. All the nurses know how much she is suffering."

Many factors influence nurses' judgments about the degree of suffering experienced by patients. One variable is the nature of the illness or injury. As the result of a nurse's experiences, both personal and professional, different illnesses or injuries become associated in a nurse's mind with different degrees of suffering. In the case of Ms. Rena and Ms. Kent, the nurses who were interviewed felt that cosmetic surgery, no matter how distressful to the patient, simply couldn't be as painful as second-degree burns. The two conditions had different meanings for the nurses. Their attitudes reflected personal judgments about pain associated with elective cosmetic surgery, and pain as a result of surgery that was required as the result of an accident.

In other instances, beliefs may be influenced by personal experiences. One nurse told us that for years, whenever a patient with a broken ankle had to be taken care of, the nurse gave the individual care and consideration, but could not possibly feel a broken ankle was as painful or as distressful as many other illnesses and injuries. "I felt a lot different about a broken ankle when I was recuperating from one. It took months. I have never been so miserable about anything as much as I was about that ankle."

Other nurses reported that illnesses and injuries took on different meanings for them as a result of their professional experience. "After awhile in practice, I got to thinking that some illnesses were really painful; others less so. I remember, when I was a nursing student, the first time I was on duty in the emergency room. A patient came in with a bad headache and complained because he had to wait two hours to see a doctor. I was all upset—two hours—the man was in dreadful pain. I think back about how naive I was. A headache is nothing compared to what we've had to handle—patients with real pain—accident victims, or whatever."

The purpose of this study was to investigate nurses' beliefs about the degree of suffering associated with various illnesses and injuries. We compiled a list of eighty illnesses and injuries nurses routinely encounter in general hospital practice. Resource people who suggested possible illnesses and injuries to be included in the list were directors of nursing, staff nurses, head nurses, and supervisors. On our final list, we could not include every illness or injury; our aim was to prepare a list of conditions consistent with the common experience of nurses in a typical urban hospital. The final list included, for example, intractable angina, second- and third-degree burns that required grafting, meningitis, coronary thrombosis, leukemia, hepatitis, hypertension, and multiple sclerosis.

We gave the list to a large group of professional nurses with various backgrounds, ages, and years of experience, and asked the nurses to rate the degree of physical pain and the degree of psychological distress they believed were associated with each illness, injury, or condition. No patient information was provided.

Findings

In general, nurses tended to infer a greater degree of psychological distress than physical pain in evaluating the suffering associated with most illnesses or injuries. For example, among the illnesses and conditions rated most painful were: intractable angina, second- and third-degree burns of upper arm and chest that require grafting, second- and third-degree burns of anterior trunk and both legs, and broken neck. For each of these, despite very high pain ratings, the ratings for psychological distress were greater than those for physical pain.

Although the nurses we studied believed that patients generally suffered more psychological distress than physical pain, the degree of psychological distress did not consistently parallel the degree of pain inferred. For example, two illnesses might be seen as involving high psychological distress, but one of these illnesses might be viewed as moderately painful. Thus, the amount of pain associated with a particular illness and injury does not determine the amount of psychological distress nurses infer for that illness or injury. This suggests that nurses do not view pain itself as a principal cause of psychological distress, but that the other characteristics of an illness or injury, such as the threat of death or long-term disability, are probably seen as sources of psychological suffering.

Physical illness or injuries seen as psychologically very distressful typically involve the threat of death or long-term, severe disability. For example, leukemia, cancer of the bladder, cancer of the breast, cancer of the uterus, and second- and third-degree burns that require extensive hospitalization were judged as psychologically very distressing.

Our most important general finding in this study was that nurses, by and large, share a common set of beliefs about the amount of pain and psychological distress associated with a variety of illnesses and injuries. The nurses we studied came from many different backgrounds and had a wide range of professional traning and experience; nevertheless, despite these personal and professional differences, their judgments about the suffering of patients with various illnesses and injuries showed a good deal of agreement. In view of these findings, one might think of beliefs about suffering as part of the *professional subculture* of nursing.

An important feature that partly defines any group that can be considered a distinct subculture is a shared set of beliefs, and the results of our research indicate that nurses do indeed share a more or less common set of beliefs about patients' suffering. To a large extent, this sharing of beliefs probably reflects common experiences that nurses have, regardless of their differing backgrounds. One nurse might specialize in pediatric care, another in obstetrics, and a third in medical-surgical nursing. But in the course of their training and professional careers, they are likely to share enough common experiences to develop a shared set of beliefs about the suffering experienced by patients with various illnesses or injuries.

In addition, nurses also teach each other the beliefs they come to share. By *teaching,* we don't mean a formal kind of instruction that we usually associate with school, but rather the kind of informal teaching and learning that occurs every day, when we share our experiences with one another. For example, a nurse who cares for a patient with pre-infarction angina talks with other nurses about the pain, as well as the psychological distress, this patient is experiencing. In this sense, then, the nurse is teaching others on the basis of this individual experience, and as a result of mutual teaching of this sort, nurses develop a shared set of beliefs.

This kind of informal teaching is an important and often valuable part of every nurse's professional education. As a consequence of sharing experiences, nurses broaden the range of one another's professional competencies. Even though a nurse may not previously have cared for a patient with a pre-infarction angina, by virtue of this sharing of experiences with other nurses, the nurse will have some expectations about the pain and psychological distress such a patient is likely to suffer. This is clearly an advantage derived from the nurse's participation in the subculture of nursing.

While recognizing the potential advantages of the shared beliefs that are part of the nursing subculture, it is also important to appreciate the fact that patients do not necessarily share this subculture. From the patient's perspective, the degree of pain or psychological distress experienced may be quite different from the level of suffering that nurses assume to be associated with the patient's particular illness. In the system of beliefs that nurses share, a draining abscess of the foot is not associated with a very high level of psychological distress. Nevertheless, for a particular patient, this condition may be exceedingly threatening and evoke a great deal of anxiety. Thus, nurses' beliefs can serve to sensitize an individual nurse to the suffering a patient is likely to experience, but special care must be taken to make sure that these beliefs do not interfere with the nurse's accurate perception of an individual patient. The beliefs shared by nurses are an important and potentially valuable part of their professional subculture, but in the final analysis, it is the nurse's understanding of the individual patient that is crucial in determining the quality of nursing care provided.

5

A Comparison of
Black and White Nurses' Judgments
about Patient Suffering

"If a patient needs me—needs my help—it doesn't matter whether that patient is black or white. My job is to help patients, not skin colors."

"It's unreal to think I feel differently about how much suffering a person has because of skin color. What I mean is, if a black patient has a broken leg, and in the next bed there's a white patient with a broken leg, I don't think to myself, 'this is a broken white leg and this is a broken black leg.' They're both broken legs."

Without exception, nurses we interviewed, regardless of their skin color, were emphatic in their statements that skin color did not affect their judgments about patient suffering. However, a number of nurses said that occasionally patients reacted to them on the basis of their racial backgrounds. A black nurse told the following account of an incident, which occurred in a hospital where this nurse had been employed for fifteen years:

"I had just gone to work in this hospital. When I took the job, I didn't ask were the patients white or black. That thought never entered my mind. I walked into the first patient's room. The patient was a white woman. I said, 'Hello.' There wasn't an answer. I introduced myself, and still she lay there without saying a word. I went about my business, continuing to make a few comments. She sat up in bed and pointed her finger at me. 'I don't want a black nurse.' I stood there for a moment. Then I caught myself getting angry, and so I waited a few more seconds before replying. I kept my voice low—purposefully low—and I told her, 'I don't care if you're orange, pink, yellow, black, or green. You're my patient. I care about the kind of job I'm going to do for you. That's what counts for me.' She didn't say a word back to me.''

A white nurse related the following experience, which occurred on a medical-surgical unit: "I went in to take care of this patient—a black man about 40 years of age. Before I got into the room, he shouted at me, 'I don't want a white nurse. I want a black nurse. You couldn't know how I feel.' '' For a moment, the nurse was taken aback. "And then I told him that I had been a nurse on that medical floor for eight years. I had every kind of color of patient in the world. I was there to help him with his ulcers, not his skin color.''

The influence of skin color on attitudes has at times given rise to a variety of beliefs. For example, some people believe that nurses of one skin color are more sensitive or empathic than nurses of another skin color. Others have maintained that black nurses feel different toward white patients than toward black patients, and white nurses have different feelings about white patient suffering than they do about black patients. Because of these biases or prejudices, we felt it important to investigate systematically the question of whether skin color affects nurses' attitudes about patient suffering, and whether, indeed, black and white nurses differed from each other in their sensitivity to patient pain and psychological distress.

Our study investigated several questions. The first was: Do black and white nurses differ in their inferences of physical pain and psychological distress? That is, when black and white nurses are asked to evaluate pain and distress in patients, will the black nurses' judgments about the degree of suffering patients are experiencing differ from those of the white nurses?

A second set of equally important questions was: Do black nurses differentially evaluate the suffering of black and white patients? Do white nurses differentially evaluate the suffering of black and white patients? Does a white nurse, for example, who has two patients of the same sex, the same age, and with the same diagnosis, view their suffering differently, simply because one is black and the other white? Does a black nurse in the identical situation have separate judgments—one for the black patient and one for the white patient—with respect to degree of suffering experienced by that patient?

Findings

The results of the study were striking: There was little difference between black and white nurses and how they rate patients' physical pain. That is, overall, both black and white nurses felt that the patients described in the questionnaire had mild or moderate pain. The racial background of the patient did not appear to influence the nurses' judgments. Black nurses judged black patients very much the same way that they judged white patients. This was also true for white nurses judging black or white patients. Black nurses, however, in comparison to white nurses, inferred greater psychological distress in patients, regardless of whether the patients were black or white. In general, therefore, when black nurses were asked to judge patients' psychological distress, they inferred greater distress than did white nurses judging the identical group of patients.

A particularly important fact is that the race of the patient did not influence the nurses' judgments. Black nurses, in comparison to white nurses, saw greater psychological distress, regardless of whether the patient was black or white. White nurses saw less psychological distress, regardless of whether the patient was black or white. The race of the nurse appeared to be the crucial factor, *not* the race of the patient.

The results of our study provide clear evidence supporting the nurses' statements that the race of the patient did not make a difference in their attitudes. The black patient who feels that a white nurse will feel different toward a black than a black nurse will is perhaps making a biased guess that is quite at variance with reality. The white nurse who told us that the race of the patient didn't concern her when it came to judging suffering was stating a fact that was true for many nurses. Of course, there may be exceptions, and you may have encountered these exceptions. But one must always guard against generalizations made on the basis of isolated cases. In general, the patient's race simply did not enter into the judgments made by either black or white nurses.

We certainly cannot presume to answer the larger question raised by the finding that black nurses tended to rate greater psychological distress in all patients than did white nurses. Does this mean that black nurses are more sensitive to or more concerned with psychological aspects of illness? Are there factors in the black American culture that sensitize the black nurse to psychological distress? We cannot answer these questions on the basis of our study, and further investigations should be undertaken to deal with these important issues.

Perhaps our most important finding, however, is that, in general, the race of the patient doesn't make a difference in nurses' judgments about patient suffering. Racial tensions may exist in hospitals, just as they do in the broader culture in which nurses live. However, some of the biased notions that have sometimes been expressed, such as the belief expressed by a patient that nurses behave differently toward patients on the basis of their skin color, must be questioned. Other factors may play a role in nurses' attitudes toward a given patient, but on the basis of the results of our study, we can conclude that the race of the patient is not a critical variable. For the majority of nurses, black patients and white patients are primarily patients, and not primarily blacks or whites. Regardless of the tensions that may operate within a given institution, or in the larger society, most nurses do not judge patients on the basis of color alone. The significance of this finding cannot be overemphasized, for it suggests that in a very important way, in their professional role, nurses transcend problems of racial prejudice.

6

Nurses' Individual Differences
and Their Effects on Judgments
of Patient Suffering

One afternoon on the maternity floor, we heard a woman ask the attending nurse if she had any children. Without waiting for an answer, the patient continued, "I wonder, because every time I complain how terrible I feel you tell me the pain isn't all that bad. I thought if you had a baby, maybe you'd know how awful I felt."

Is it necessary for nurses to have personally experienced physical suffering in order to empathize with patients' expressions of pain? There were a number of reactions when we discussed this incident with a group of nurses. One nurse agreed with the patient. She said that for several years she had worked as an obstetrical nurse. "A couple of us who didn't have children at the time thought some of the women exaggerated their discomfort. No matter what we did, there were always a few who carried on like they were dying. I know we thought they were putting on a show for attention. Then I had my first baby and had a terrible time. I won't go into the details, but now that I'm back at work, when a woman starts telling me how miserable she is, I believe her. I know because of what I went through; my attitude changed."

Other nurses voiced opposite points of view. " I don't think it's necessary for me to have suffered in order to be sympathetic," said one nurse. "I had easy deliveries. This doesn't mean I can't sympathize with women who have a rough time. I judge each situation. I can tell from the way a patient looks, what she says, how she responds to me whether she's really in pain or just demanding attention.''

One underlying premise behind our research is that we can never directly observe the suffering of another person. In the case of patients, pain and distress is within that patient. The most a nurse can do is observe the patient and, on the basis of cues, make a judgment about how much physical pain and psychological distress that person is experiencing. In our other studies, we have investigated characteristics of patients that affect nurses' judgments. For example, the age, social class, ethnic background, sex, and nature of the illness or injury of the patient were characteristics that influenced nurses' judgments of patient suffering. The purpose of this study, however, was to look at some characteristics of nurses that might affect the inferences made about patient suffering.

Observations of nurses, folklore of nursing, and general psychological theory suggested a number of variables worth exploring. For example, does the fact that an individual nurse has personally experienced a good deal of pain and distress contribute toward that nurse's inference of a relatively high degree of pain in others who are ill or injured? Similarly, if one has experienced considerable psychological distress in one's own life, does the experience make the person more sensitive to the psychological distress in others? In the preceding example, a number of nurses believed personal experiences with childbirth increased their sympathies for maternity patients who experienced difficulty in labor. Others disagreed.

Another variable we considered important to investigate is a commonly held notion that, as a result of repeated experiences with people in pain and distress, a nurse might become less sensitive.

"I realized after I started to work how sheltered I had been in nursing school," one nurse reported. "We never really saw patients who were suffering. It was pretty hard for me when I first began to work after graduation. The first weeks I was drained. I couldn't take the pain and suffering. I didn't think I was going to last as a nurse. I had friends who felt the same way. But we stayed, and the first shock wore off. We got used to seeing suffering. I don't think I really felt less—I'm not sure though—but after awhile, something that would have shocked me no longer bothered me. When you see patients suffering day after day, you can't help but adapt. Now, something has to be terribly serious before I take it to heart the way I did my first year."

A contrary point of view was expressed by another nurse. "I haven't changed from the first day I started to work. I felt I was sheltered from patient suffering in school, but working has only made me more aware than before how real suffering is. If anything, I find myself much more sensitive as time goes on. I'm much more aware. I don't see how anyone who works day after day, year after year, seeing people suffer can help but feel more and more aware of what it means to be a patient."

Given these differing opinions, it would seem important to investigate how the varying lengths of nurses' working experience influence their judgments of patient suffering.

Another important variable we considered is the type of position a nurse holds. Staff nurses have frequently told us that a nurse who isn't involved directly in patient care can't possibly understand either patient or staff problems. On the other hand, supervisors and administrators have denied this assertion, maintaining that a nurse who moves into a position with more administrative responsibilities doesn't necessarily lose touch, either with staff or with patients.

Just as the type of position might affect nurses' judgments, we also wondered whether nurses' areas of specialization would affect their perceptions. Would a nurse who works on a psychiatric unit, for example, be more sensitive to psychological distress than to physical pain? Conversely, would a nurse working in an area where there is a great deal of physical pain—for example, the intensive care unit—be more aware of physical pain than psychological distress?

And finally, national or ethnic background represented another variable to examine. It is commonly assumed that people from Anglo-Saxon, Germanic, and Scandinavian backgrounds tend to be somewhat more stoic in their attitudes toward pain and psychological distress in comparison to those from Mediterranean and some other cultural or ethnic backgrounds. Obviously this reflects certain stereotyped beliefs about national, ethnic, or cultural differences. However, because such stereotypes often have little basis in fact, national and ethnic backgrounds of nurses seemed important to consider in this exploratory study.

Participants in the study included nurses from all specialty areas and administrative positions. Their professional experience ranged in length from one year to forty years. The majority were born in the United States, with over fifty coming from North European backgrounds, and the remainder representing other ethnic groups.

The subjects were given the *Standard Measure of Inferences of Suffering* questionnaire, consisting of sixty items describing patients with a variety of illnesses or conditions (see Appendix). The nurses also filled out a questionnaire rating their own experiences with pain, personal data, and several other psychological scales dealing with their stoicism, preferences for interpersonal or technical duties, and so forth.

Findings

The nurses' ratings of their own pain were directly related to their ratings of pain in others. That is, nurses who tended to infer high degrees of physical pain in patients also reported more painful experiences in their own lives. Conversely, nurses who rated relatively low physical pain in patients reported various personal experiences as less painful. In other words, nurses rated their patients' pain to be similar to their own.

Judgments about the amount of one's own psychological distress experienced were not significantly related to judgments about the psychological distress in patients. There was some relationship, however, between the amount of psychological distress nurses inferred in patients and their tendency to prefer interpersonal aspects of nursing. Nurses who tended to infer relatively high suffering in patients also tended to prefer those aspects of nursing that concerned relating to their patients, while those who inferred less suffering preferred the more technical aspects of nursing.

A very interesting finding of this study was that the ages, experience, and positions of the nurses were *not* related to judgments of patient pain and distress. That is, there were older nurses who inferred considerable pain in patients and younger nurses who reacted the same way. There were both young nurses and older nurses who inferred little suffering. Just as the ages and experience of the nurses did not influence inferences, the positions nurses held were unrelated to the kinds of inferences made about patient suffering. Some administrators judged considerable suffering; others inferred relatively low degrees of suffering. Similarly, staff nurses and supervisors also varied. The generalization sometimes heard—that individuals in supervisor positions, far removed from direct patient care, tend to be less empathic—simply doesn't seem to be valid. The individual nurse and not the nurse's position is what determines a nurse's judgments.

Although the nurses' ages, experience, and types of position were not related to their inferences of patient suffering, we did find that ethnic and/or national backgrounds were important determinants of their beliefs about pain and psychological distress. The sample of nurses was divided into two groups, one group from North European backgrounds (English, German, Scandinavian, and so forth) and the other from East European, South European, and African backgrounds. The results showed that nurses with African, South European, or East European backgrounds inferred relatively high patient suffering, while nurses from North European backgrounds inferred relatively less suffering. Although there were exceptions to this general finding, it was largely the nurses whose family backgrounds were Italian, Polish, Russian, Spanish, or African who judged patients to be suffering the most pain, and the nurses with English, Irish, German, or Scandinavian family backgrounds who judged patients to suffer the least.

Insofar as pain is concerned, our findings indicate that nurses who are generally very sensitive to patients' pain also report, with some exceptions, that they have had some rather painful experiences in their own lives.

This finding has certain implications for the training of nurses.

It certainly does *not* mean that nurses have to suffer themselves in order to empathize with the suffering of their patients. But it does suggest that in one way or another, a nurse should learn about the experience of pain. Personal experience with pain is only one way in which this can be achieved. We also learn from the experience of others if we pay attention to these experiences, if we listen to what others say, and if we read what others have written. For example, people who have suffered a great deal of pain, as a result of illness, injury, or some other circumstances, have written about their experiences, and reading these reports can serve as a very effective way of learning about other people's feelings. Similarly, as part of a nurses education, it may be important for her to devote a certain amount of time to exploring patients' experiences, finding out in detail how they are feeling. Probably most, if not all, nurses do this as part of their training, but it may be worthwhile to introduce this kind of exploration of patients' feelings as a regular, systematic part of training throughout a nurses's professional education.

Our findings with regard to differences among nurses of various ethnic and national backgrounds fit in with the common observation that some cultures tend to be more stoic about suffering than other cultures. Each of us learns how to interpret our experiences on the basis of our interactions with others as we are growing up. Therefore, a person growing up among people who usually discount or minimize feelings of pain or psychological distress will be likely to learn to be relatively stoic in judging suffering. And those who grow up among people who emphasize or maximize suffering are likely to learn the same pattern of responses themselves.

There is no right or wrong in this matter. It is not necessarily better or worse to grow up in a culture that tends to be either very stoic or very sensitive to pain. But it is extremely important for nurses to recognize the influence of their own cultural backgrounds on their judgments about patients' experiences. A nurse whose background differs markedly from that of a patient may not intuitively empathize with the patient's experience. But the nurse *can* more fully understand the patient if the patient's background and the ways in which the nurse has learned to interpret painful experiences are both taken into account. A nurse, for example, who has grown up in a culture that has fostered a stoic attitude toward pain may not respond with intuitive empathy to a patient whose culture tends to emphasize reactions to pain. Nevertheless, the nurse who is aware of these attitudes toward pain can be more accurate in understanding a patient's feelings by taking these attitudes into account.

7

How Nurses from
Different Cultural Backgrounds
View Patient Suffering

In Bangkok, Thailand, a 42-year-old Thai man has bronchopneumonia. When he is admitted to the hospital, Thai nurses attend to his needs. In Pusan, Korea, a Korean man about the same age is hospitalized for the identical condition. Korean nurses act to alleviate his pain and distress. Somewhere in the United States, an American man in his early 40s is rushed to the hospital with the identical diagnosis. American nurses on the staff care for this patient.

Events of a similar nature occur in every part of the world every day. A child who is stricken with meningitis, for example, in Japan, Belgium, England, or Nepal, is hospitalized. Nurses native to that culture care for him. Yet, nurses in every society share common professional goals: specifically, to meet patients' needs by responding to their pain and psychological distress.

Although nurses from very different cultural backgrounds have similar objectives, do they hold common beliefs about suffering? We are all aware that each culture has its own set of customs and values. For example, one culture may place a high value on stoicism. For people in that culture to show emotions is not considered acceptable. A

We wish to express our appreciation to the American Nurses' Foundation and the International Communications Network of the American Nurses' Foundation for their interest in and financial support of the cross-cultural studies.

brave attitude is respected; tears may be for the weak. If one runs into difficulty and has discomfort, the suffering must be kept hidden from the rest of society. One has a public face; emotions of any sort remain concealed behind the mask of a smiling expression. Yet, in another culture, expressiveness is the accepted way for people to respond to life's fortunes or misfortunes. One shows one's feelings. There will be tears and cries if there is tragedy; there will be laughter and smiles for occasions of pleasure.

The way we learn to behave depends, in part, on the culture in which we are born and raised. Often we are not even aware of how much our behavior is influenced by the culture in which we live. Only when we visit another culture are we aware of the different behavioral responses to the same phenomena. The response to death of families in the United States had surprised a nurse from Nigeria, for example. In this nurse's home country, death was not feared. The death of a family member was a sad event, of course, because it meant the loss of a loved one; however, the mourning period was also an occasion for celebration. There would be gatherings of all the clan with feasts for singing. The nurse's mother had her burial clothes in readiness. She regularly washed and cleaned the garments. A strong belief in an afterlife cast a positive glow over their view of death and dying. Death was viewed not as an end, but as a beginning.

Since cultures differ in customs, values, and ways of perceiving and interpreting various phenomena, we might expect nurses from various cultures to differ in their inferences of suffering associated with illnesses or injuries. In one of our past studies, entitled "Foreign and American Nurses: Reactions and Interactions," we found that differences in cultural attitudes led to some misunderstandings among colleagues.[1] One American nurse was annoyed when a foreign nurse continually told her how callous American nurses were towards elderly patients.

"She said that we had no respect for old people. In her country, anyone past 60 was held in a revered position. Old people were never

[1]Lois J. Davitz, J. R. Davitz, and Yasuko Sameshima, "Foreign and American Nurses: Reactions and Interactions," *Nursing Outlook,* April 1976.

left alone. The families always made sure old people had a place to live, plenty to eat, and the companionship of children and grand-children. I don't think she is being fair. I know that after I talked to her about her family, I felt she was the one who was callous—not about old people, but young.''

The foreign nurse referred to had left her four children between the ages of 5 and 12 in the care of her husband while she came to the United States to work. She had not returned to her native land for three years and had no plans to return in the immediate future. Her in-tention was to complete an advanced degree and obtain several years of work experience before going back to her family.

"She wasn't one to talk about us being neglectful of old people. What about her own children?''

The foreign nurse saw the situation quite differently. In her country, children were raised not only by parents but by an extended family.

"Our children are very close to parents. This doesn't mean the parents have to spend every day with them. My children know I am here to study and to work. I write them very often. The two eldest will be coming over to live with me next month. We will all go back together. My husband understands that it is important for me to finish my work here.''

In another instance, a nurse from a culture that placed a high value on males was criticized by American nurses. The head nurse, an American, noted that the nurse was marvelous with male patients.

"She'll do anything they ask her to do. With women, it's another story. She'll do the minimum.''

For the nurse from a culture that evaluates women as secon-dary to males, behaving differently toward females was not being un-fair or insensitive. Her behavior merely reflected a cultural orienta-tion.

This nurse believed that women do not have as much pain as males. "Women can stand pain. They do not hurt as much. That's why it is necessary to do more for men. They need more.''

A middle-aged male who had been injured in an automobile accident was brought into the emergency room of a large metropolitan hospital. Accustomed to crises, the staff responded quickly and efficiently. After the patient was transferred to the medical-surgical unit, we talked about the case with the nurses who had been on duty at that time. An American nurse expressed surprise that the man was so emotional. "I'm used to men holding back their feelings. I could have understood the behavior if he had been a kid. I always feel that with children it's much harder when they're hurt. They don't know what's happening to them. Kids' suffering really bothers me. But this man wasn't all that serious, and he should have realized there was no need to carry on as if he were dying."

Several other nurses from North European backgrounds who had recently immigrated to the United States agreed. "Where I come from," one told us, "we never want other people to know we feel bad about something."

This nurse could remember that, as a child, when any children in the family were hurt, they were first told not to cry. "My mother would say 'you're too big to cry.' The only times I can recall being spanked were for crying. That man's crying surprised me."

A Puerto Rican nurse disagreed. "The man was emotional," she said, "but he was worried about himself and his wife. I don't blame him for being upset. I would have acted the same way—my husband, too. I can remember when my daughter was hurt riding her bicycle. My husband carried on worse than she."

For some nurses, stoicism and self-control are expected in the face of suffering; for other nurses, giving way to feelings is accepted as perfectly normal and acceptable. What appears to make a difference in the reactions these nurses give is their cultural orientation. All of the nurses were experienced professionals with the same goals concerning patient care. However, their attitudes toward the suffering of the patients differed as a result of their cultural backgrounds.

In an effort to answer the question of whether cultural differences affect nurses' judgments about patient suffering, we decided to investigate nurses' attitudes within various cultures. Clearly, we would not expect all nurses from one culture to think alike; however, our objective was to find out if nurses from one culture shared a common belief system and if this belief system was different from that of other cultures.

The overall question we raised was: Do nurses from different cultures infer different degrees of suffering in the same patients? For example, in caring for a Japanese man with bleeding ulcers, would a Japanese nurse infer degrees of suffering in the patient different from a Belgian nurse caring for a Belgian man with the same symptoms? Would a Nigerian nurse working with a child with a fractured femur infer different degrees of suffering from those inferred by a Korean nurse caring for a Korean child with the identical condition?

This study, which took over three years to complete, involved the cooperation of about one thousand nurses from the following countries: United States, Uganda, Belgium, Thailand, Japan, Nigeria, Nepal, Formosa (Taiwan), England, Korea, Israel, India, and Puerto Rico. It should be noted that Puerto Rican nurses, although citizens of the United States, voluntarily suggested that they be considered separately from nurses born and raised within the continental United States. All the nurses, who varied in age, experience, and specialty, were licensed and professionally employed in their respective cultures.

The instrument used in this study was the *Standard Measure of Inferences of Suffering* questionnaire developed for many of the studies reported in this book. Included in the questionnaire were sixty descriptions of male and female patients with a variety of illnesses or conditions. Each item had two scales, one for physical pain and another for psychological distress. The task for the nurses in each country was to read the descriptions of the patients and, on the basis of their own judgments, rate each patient in terms of the degree of physical pain or psychological distress they felt the patient experienced. As in all the studies, the nurses were explicitly told there were no right or wrong answers. We were only interested in their opinions. This was not a test. We were concerned with the kinds of judgments nurses made about suffering.

The English version of the questionnaire was distributed to nurses in the United States, England, India, Uganda, and Nigeria. The nurses in all five of these countries are fluent in English, the common language of these lands. The only substantive change made in the questionnaire used in India, Nigeria, and Uganda was the omission of first names and surnames for the hypothetical cases. Patients were simply designated as male or female. The reason for this change was to eliminate possible bias. In India, Nigeria, and Uganda, names may indicate tribal, caste, or social class affiliation.

Preparation of the questionnaires in the other languages was a major undertaking involving three steps. First, bilingual nurses translated the English questionnaire into French, Chinese, Hebrew, Japanese, Korean, Nepalese, Spanish, and Thai. The translated questionnaires were given to another group of bilingual nurses for translation back into English. A third group of bilingual nurses compared the two translated English versions. Questionnaires in each of the languages were then prepared for duplication. In some instances, because of the unavailability of typewriters—for example, Chinese, Japanese, and Korean typewriters—it was necessary to hand-letter a master copy. The questionnaires for each country were sent to nurse leaders who had volunteered to serve as liaisons for this study. Their responsibilities included contacting hospitals, arranging for volunteer subjects, distributing the questionnaires, and returning the completed questionnaires to the authors in the United States.

Figure 1 shows how one question appeared in the different languages.

Findings

This study began with the assumption that nurses' attitudes about suffering are, in part, socially learned responses. The results incontrovertibly confirm this assumption. Nurses from one culture markedly differed from nurses from another culture in their inferences of physical pain and psychological distress. The data in the study were collected within each culture. The patient descriptions were identical, and yet

Figure 1. Question #7 in Different Languages

ENGLISH

	None	Little	Mild	Mod-erate	Great	Severe	Very Severe
7. After a series of tests and examinations, Catherine Kent, forty-two years of age, was hospitalized with thrombophlebitis. Therapeutic measures include anticoagulants and bedrest.							
Physical Pain, Discomfort:	1	2	3	4	5	6	7
Psychological Distress:	1	2	3	4	5	6	7

HEBREW

שאלון | בכאב | בצער | בחרדה | או במצוקה | באיזו מידה

כאב־פיזי, אי־נוחיות:	1	2	3	4	5	6	7
מצוקה נפשית:	1	2	3	4	5	6	7

7. לאחר סדרת בדיקות ואבחונים, אושפזה קתרין קנט, בת ארבעים ושתיים, עם דלקת ורידים. האמצעים הטיפוליים כוללים תרופות נגד קרישה ומנוחה במיטה.

JAPANESE

7. 一通りの検査の結果、42才のアン・ケリーさんは静脈血管血栓症と診断され入院させられた。治療法は安静等と抗凝固剤の投薬である。

肉体的 苦痛	1	2	3	4	5	6	7
精神的 苦しみ	1	2	3	4	5	6	7

Figure 1 (continued)

CHINESE

7. 康太太七七歲，在經過各項
測驗及×光檢查後診斷，
其為血栓性靜脈炎，故
住院接受抗凝血劑藥物
治療及臥床休息。

身體方面
之疼痛，　1　2　3　4　5　6　7
不舒服：

心理方　　1　2　3　4　5　6　7
面之不安：

NEPALESE

　　　शारीरिक ×　२　3　8　५　६　७
पीडा तथा
बेचैनी

मानसिक ×　२　3　8　५　६　७
पीडा

FRENCH

7. A la suite d'une série de tests et
d'examens, Catherine Iseri, âgée de
quarante deux ans, a été hospitalisée
pour thrombophlébite. Les mesures
thérapeutiques comprennent anticoag-
ulant et repos au lit.

Douleur
Physique ou　1　2　3　4　5　6　7
Malaise

Angoisse
Psychologique 1　2　3　4　5　6　7

nurses from various cultures responded differently to the same information.

Among the cultures studied, Korean nurses inferred the greatest psychological distress. Puerto Rican nurses were the second highest, Uganda the next. Nurses from Nepal, Taiwan, and Belgium inferred the least amount of psychological distress. The following list presents the findings in rank order; that is, the first country represents the greatest inferences of suffering and the second, the next highest, and so forth.

Inferences of psychological distress ranked from highest to lowest:
1. Korea
2. Puerto Rico
3. Japan
4. Uganda
5. India
6. Nigeria
7. United States
8. Thailand
9. England
10. Israel
11. Belgium
12. Taiwan (Formosa)
13. Nepal

Among the cultures included in this study, Korean nurses inferred the greatest amount of physical pain for the patients described in the questionnaire. Japanese nurses were second and Indian nurses third. Nurses from Belgium, the United States, and England inferred the least amount of physical pain. The following list presents the rank order of each of the countries with regard to inferences of physical pain.

Inferences of physical pain ranked from highest to lowest:
1. Korea
2. Japan

3. India
4. Uganda
5. Nepal
6. Taiwan (Formosa)
7. Nigeria
8. Israel
9. Thailand
10. Puerto Rico
11. Belgium
12. United States
13. England

An important implication of this study is the appreciation and recognition of markedly different cultural responses to inferences of physical pain and psychological distress. It is interesting to note that Korean and Japanese nurses inferred both great physical pain and psychological distress, particularly in view of the fact that many people in western societies think of these oriental groups as stoic and less sensitive to suffering. In our study concerned with ethnic backgrounds of patients, American nurses, for example, rated Japanese and Korean patients as having little pain or distress. However, when Japanese and Korean nurses rated Japanese and Korean patients, the perception of suffering was quite different.

According to a Japanese colleague, Westerners cannot "read" Japanese people. She stated that, "as little children, we are taught not to show feelings on our faces. We will smile for the world, but inside we may feel great despair."

The differences among Korean, Japanese, Thai, Chinese, and Nepalese nurses were striking. When we presented these findings to a group of nurses, one comment was, "Weren't you really comparing oriental and western societies?" For this nurse, and for some Westerners, oriental people are part of one group. The results of this study demonstrate that oriental national groups differ among themselves, just as one would expect groups from various western societies to differ. In America, these differences aren't always recognized, and there is a tendency to stereotype the stoic Oriental.

Among the cultures studied, the Nepalese and Chinese nurses consistently inferred the lowest amount of psychological distress. We talked with Nepalese nurses and Chinese nurses in the United States about this finding. In their view, there is much less emphasis placed in their cultures on interpretations of feelings. One Nepalese nurse noted, for example, that in Nepal the study of psychology of behavior and motivations for nurses was certainly not prominent in the curriculum. A Chinese nurse believed that Chinese people did not have the inner "turmoil" the nurse felt many Americans seemed to experience. The explanation offered by the Chinese nurse was quite different from that of the Japanese nurse, who stated that, whereas children are taught to inhibit overt expressions of distress, at the same time, intensity of emotional experiences and sensitivity of feelings on an experiential level were highly valued in Japanese families.

The Puerto Rican nurses rated psychological distress of patients very high and physical pain very low. Obviously, our data cannot explain this finding, but we might share the interpretations that several Puerto Rican nurses offered.

"We know our people are very emotional. We are always expressing what we feel—singing, dancing, laughter—so if someone is in the hospital, we know they feel very upset, but they might not have much pain. When I take care of a Puerto Rican patient, I expect them to tell me how terrible they feel. They do feel bad, no matter what is wrong with them. Just because they complain a lot, I know they might not really be in pain. I am used to Puerto Rican people being very dramatic about themselves."

It is particularly interesting to look at the ratings of Jewish nurses for Jewish patients in Israel. Relatively low degrees of suffering for both physical pain and psychological distress were inferred. In our study of American nurses' beliefs about the suffering of patients from different ethnic backgrounds, the American nurses judged Jewish patients' suffering among the highest of any ethnic group. In interviews with American nurses from non-Jewish backgrounds, the nurses revealed that they felt that Jewish patients are more demanding and express their suffering more than any other group of people.

However, this contrasts sharply with the opinions of Israeli nurses dealing with Israeli patients.

The samples from Belgium, the United States, and England gave the lowest ratings for physical pain, rating psychological distress about equally. English nurses, among all the cultures, were the lowest for physical pain. According to some researchers, individuals from Anglo-Saxon and Germanic backgrounds tend to curtail their expressions of pain. In our talks with English nurses working in the United States, we were repeatedly told that one of their major adjustments to patients had been the fact that people in America had such little tolerance for pain. They talked about English patients having resiliency and strength. As one told us, "British people do keep a stiff upper lip." Certainly, in terms of our findings, British nurses infer little pain in patients and not much more psychological distress.

The findings from this study provide dramatic evidence of the importance of one's point of view in making inferences about another person's experiences. The results also raise important questions about relationships of nurses with patients. If nurses from one culture hold a particular set of beliefs about another culture, do these beliefs influence the quality and nature of the care they give? To what degree does stereotyping of another culture influence professional practice?

There are important implications of this study for American nurses who, perhaps more than nurses in the other cultures studied, come into regular contact with people from various ethnic backgrounds. Our interviews with nurses revealed innumerable instances where they found themselves reacting strongly to what they felt were unwarranted reactions to situations. For example, how do the beliefs of nurses from Anglo-Saxon or Germanic backgrounds, who tend to minimize physical pain and psychological distress, as our findings indicate, influence their treatment of individuals from Korean or Japanese backgrounds? The external behavior of these people might not indicate the depth of their feelings. Thus, meaningful relationships between nurses and patients are blocked, simply because of vast differences in cultural orientations.

We certainly do not propose that nurses discard their belief systems and become "universalists" in their thinking. We do suggest, however, that through nurses' understanding of their own belief systems about suffering, the cultural patterns that are part of their thinking can provide them with insights that will help nurses to deal effectively with patients whose values and attitudes differ from their own. An important consequence of the recognition of cultural differences in beliefs about suffering can prevent a great deal of misunderstanding and misconceptions, and can lead to more effective, sensitive patient care.

8
Observations of
Nurse-Patient Interaction
in Hospital Settings

Do behaviors reflect feelings? For example, if we feel a patient is experiencing considerable pain or distress, will we behave differently than we would for another patient whom we believe isn't suffering?

"This certainly is the case with me," one nurse told us. "People always tell me they can tell exactly what I feel by the way I talk and what I do. I think most people can only go so far in controlling themselves. I'll have a patient who I think is really suffering. Maybe all the patient needs is me to stand there holding the patient's hand, talking about the weather or the patient's family—whatever. It doesn't matter to me how many times that patient calls; I want to do something.

"But take some patients who I know aren't in pain. Like the one I had who must have called for a nurse twenty times one day. Not one request had anything to do with pain or being uncomfortable. The patient wanted a maid, not a nurse."

We began this research with the assumption that most students who enter nursing training are especially sensitive to the pain and distress of others. In our interviews with nursing students about why they had chosen nursing careers, one of the major factors revealed was a desire to alleviate suffering. For some people, however, the day-to-day experience working with suffering patients can be personally upsetting. As a result, these individuals develop mechanisms that help maintain psychological distance between themselves and their patients' suffering.

"I think you learn after awhile *not* to feel," one nurse told us. "I know that if I felt all my patients were really suffering a great deal, I couldn't last a day. I'd be emotionally drained. I'd probably leave nursing, and I think I'm a good nurse. I don't want to minimize the suffering of patients, but in my experience some people make a big thing out of something minor. Like the patient we had on the floor last week with an abscess on the foot. I'm not saying this patient wasn't uncomfortable, but I can't believe the pain was as bad as it was made out to be."

One way this nurse achieved psychological distance was to minimize pain and distress inferred about some of the patients. Through believing that the patient is "really not suffering too much," caring for that individual becomes psychologically safer.

Thus, nurses' inferences of relatively low suffering among patients may be viewed, in part, as a defensive or distancing mechanism that permits the nurse to maintain her own psychological integrity in the face of daily contact with people in pain, people who are experiencing considerable psychological distress, and people who may be dying.

Our various studies have shown that nurses have different attitudes toward patient suffering. Some nurses inferred high degrees of suffering and others, much lower degrees of suffering. In any event, if low inferences of suffering represent, at least in part, defensive mechanisms nurses use to make daily contact with pain and distress psychologically tolerable, it would be reasonable to expect similar distancing reflected in nursing behaviors.

For example, if nurses inferred high degrees of suffering in patients, we might expect these nurses to become emotionally involved with their patients and very concerned about providing the comforting aspects of patient care. And conversely, nurses who judged relatively little patient suffering would tend to distance themselves and show greater concern with the more technical aspects of care, as well as being less supportive of patient complaints.

The goal of the three studies in this part of the research was to study the relationship between nursing behaviors and inferences of suffering. One study considered nurses working in medical-surgical units; the second study focused on nurses in obstetrics; and the third study involved pediatric nurses.

Our first task was to identify two groups of nurses in each of the three settings. One group included nurses who inferred considerable suffering in patients and the other group included nurses who inferred low patient suffering. We identified these two groups of nurses in the following manner.

The *Standard Measure of Inferences of Suffering* questionnaire was given to a large number of nurses in each of the three settings. The questionnaire consisted of sixty items, each describing a patient with a given illness or injury. The volunteer subjects rated these hypothetical patients on two dimensions—pain and psychological distress. Each subject received a score, and on the basis of the total scores, two groups of nurses were identified: maximizers, or high-inference nurses, and minimizers, or low-inference nurses. These two groups of individuals were contacted and asked to volunteer for the second stage of the research, which involved observations of their interactions with patients.

Permission to observe these interactions was granted by the hospitals, as well as the patients the nurses attended. On a given day, a nurse observer, wearing a nurse's uniform, accompanied a nurse from the high-inference or the low-inference group. The nurse observers were not told in which group the nurse they were observing had been assigned. The task for the observer was to remain as unobtrusive as possible. In no way was the observer to comment or interact with the patient or any other person in the unit. The observer's job was merely to observe the behaviors of the nurse, following an observation schedule that will be described later.

In this kind of research, there is always some question whether the presence of an observer affects the behavior of any of the individuals being observed. The use of nonparticipant observers in social science research is standard practice. Ideally, hidden television cameras, tape recorders, and other technical devices would provide the most objective data. Ethically, however, the use of any of these methods is not realistically possible or appropriate.

In this study, some of the nurses reported that they were aware of an observer. However, without exception, all stated that after a short period they forgot about the observer or adapted to the observer's presence. One nurse commented, for example, that "at the start, I was aware of her in the corner of the room. But then, I got so busy, I completely forgot she was there. At the end of the day, I remember being surprised to find she was still around."

In one instance, the nurse said that they were used to having lots of people around on the floor. The observer was just another "face."

Another nurse commented, "When we really get busy on the unit, I wouldn't recognize my own mother. There isn't time to look around."

In addition to being unobtrusive, the observers were instructed not to interact with the nurse being observed at any time during the day. That is, even during breaks, lunch hours, at the nurses' station, and elsewhere, the observer and the nurse did not communicate. After the observations were finished, the nurse and the observer were free to discuss the study and the observation guide.

After extensive training, the observers employed an observation schedule developed specifically for this research. In developing the schedule, several aims had to be kept in mind. First, the schedule had to provide an objective basis for obtaining reliable observations. Second, the method of recording data had to be concise and rapid enough to be usable in collecting observations of quickly occurring events. Third, the method of observing and recording had to be as unobtrusive as possible, because the use of mechanical devices, such as tape recorders, movie cameras, and so forth, were not used. Fourth, the schedule had to provide a basis for recording the range of nursing behaviors likely to occur in each of three hospital-unit settings: medical-surgical, obstetrics, and pediatrics.

The final observation schedule consisted of three major sections. The first section dealt with nurses' verbal behavior and included such categories as the following: whether the nurse being observed asked an opening question, dismissed patient's worries or concerns, gave an order or directive, replied to patient's questions, and so forth.

The second section of the observation schedule considered nurses' actions. These included, for example: gave backrub; changed dressings; gave medication; straightened bedding, fixtures, and so forth.

The third section covered nurses' relations with the patients. These categories included: physical distance, or where the nurse stood in relation to the patient; emotional tone, such as whether the nurse was irritated, withdrawn, businesslike, warm, pleasant, and so forth; and level of activity, such as the touching and gentleness shown the patient.

The observer accompanied a nurse for a given period of time on typical working shifts. Observations were recorded by checking the appropriate categories in the observation schedule.

The findings for each of the three groups—medical-surgical, pediatrics, and obstetrics—will be discussed separately.

Findings of Study One:
Medical-Surgical Nurses

Results

Before looking at the difference between the high- and low-inference nurses, we will consider the overall behavior of the entire sample of medical-surgical nurses. For verbal interactions, the most frequent category of behavior was "asks opening question," followed by "gives order," and "verbalizes, explains actions to be taken."

The following example describes what typically occurred. The patient requested to see a nurse either by putting on a call light or by using a buzzer system. The nurse entered the room and asked the patient the reason for the call. Following the patient's response, the nurse gave an order; for example, the need for the patient to change position, take medication, and so forth. If an action was taken, the nurse performed the action and, if the procedure was unfamiliar, explained the action.

Somewhat less frequent were sympathetic and reassuring replies to patients' questions. There was generally very little discussion of the patient's condition and very little exploration of patient's feelings. The response of the nurse was brief and focused on the patient's immediate complaint.

The most frequent nursing action was some form of physical nurturing and the closely related category of changing the patient's position. All the other categories of nursing actions occurred only once, suggesting that the majority of nurse-patient interactions involved verbal exchanges.

Differences between High- and Low-Inference Nurses in Medical-Surgical Settings

Verbal interactions. The findings of this study indicated that high-inference nurses behaved differently from low-inference nurses with respect to verbal interactions. Nurses who inferred relatively high degrees of suffering more often described or explained to the patients the nursing actions they had taken or were about to take. Rather than merely giving an order—for example, "Turn over on your back"—they discussed the reasons for turning over and what actions they were going to take. Nurses in the high-inference group, for example, who might be giving an injection, would introduce themselves to the patient, explain the reason for the injection, and answer any questions. Frequently, information was also provided while a procedure was being followed.

In contrast, low-inference nurses tended not to discuss their actions. For example, the statement, "I'm going to get you ready for an I.V." would not be followed with a description of the I.V. procedure and the reasons for the I.V. If a patient was being taken for tests, again the rationale for the tests was not detailed. In general, low-inference nurses gave brief replies to patients' questions, in contrast to the high-inference nurses who provided considerably more information.

When patients expressed concerns that were psychologically based, high-inference nurses made an effort to express sympathetic understanding. Low-inference nurses were much more matter-of-fact. Low-inference nurses rarely made a referral when patients expressed considerable or repeated discomfort. For example, when a high-inference nurse was unable to give an answer to a patient's question, she offered to check with other resource people, such as a doctor or supervisor. The low-inference nurses deflected the question, either avoiding a direct response or changing the subject.

Nursing actions.   A wide range of nursing actions was observed in the medical-surgical unit group. In general, the high-inference group was significantly different from the low-inference group. The high inference group engaged in many more direct actions that involved physical contact, such as helping the patient to change positions and rechecking a dressing to reassure a patient. In contrast, low-inference nurses engaged in appreciably more "straightening" behaviors, such as fixing the bedding and filling a pitcher with water, which involved little or no patient contact. Thus, low-inference nurses were more concerned with objects and equipment, while high-inference nurses focused more directly on the patient.

Nurses' relations with patients.   The high-inference group in the medical-surgical unit differed from the low-inference group in their relations with the patients. We might illustrate this through a generalized portrait of a nurse in each group. The typical high-inference nurse stood close to the patient's bed, more often than not near the head of the bed. During the conversation or question-and-answer dialogue, the high-inference nurse would reach out and touch the patient, take the patient's hand, smooth hair back from the forehead, or pat the patient's shoulder. If possible, the nurse maintained eye contact, speaking directly to the patient.

In contrast, the low-inference nurse was attentive but behaved somewhat differently. This nurse would commonly stand at the foot of the bed. On occasion, the low-inference nurse entered the doorway and addressed the patient from some distance. Rather than reaching out and touching the patient, this nurse might straighten the patient's possessions, offer to refill a water jug, or do various things that were all attentive, but did not involve physical touch of a comforting nature.

In addition to greater physical distance from the patient, the nurses who inferred relatively low levels of suffering also tended to have a more neutral or matter-of-fact emotional attitude toward the patient, touched the patient less frequently, engaged in somewhat more impersonal nursing actions, tended to dismiss patients' worries more frequently, and discussed or explained nursing actions less often. In general, nurses in the low-inference group, in comparison to those in the high-inference group, were more impersonal and distant in their interactions with patients. In short, their behavior reflected and mirrored their beliefs about patient suffering.

Findings of Study Two: Obstetric Nurses

The aim of our second study was to determine whether nurses' beliefs about suffering are related to nursing behaviors in a setting quite different from the usual medical-surgical unit. Of the many possibilities available, the obstetrics unit was chosen as one that was clearly different in many respects from the medical-surgical unit; also, it provided a setting in which nurses must frequently deal with the issue of patient's pain.

We generally expected the same findings as those in our initial study of medical-surgical nurses. That is, the tendency to infer relatively low suffering in patients was viewed primarily as a defensive mechanism, which would be reflected by nursing behaviors that increased the psychological distance between nurse and patient. Because of the difference in settings and in the kinds of demands made upon the nurse, we did not expect the results for obstetric nurses to be identical to those obtained for medical-surgical nurses; nevertheless, we did expect the same trends.

The design of this study repeated that of the initial study of medical-surgical nurses. From a large sample of obstetric nurses, a group who tended to infer relatively high patient suffering and a group who tended to infer relatively low patient suffering were identified. Interactions of nurses in these two groups with patients were observed, and their behaviors were compared in terms of verbal interactions, nursing actions, and relation to patient.

As in the preceding study, a nurse-observer accompanied each nurse in the sample, observing and recording the nurse's interactions with patients. To account for the somewhat different actions taken by obstetric nurses in comparison to those in the medical-surgical unit, the observation schedule was slightly revised. Administering an enema was added to the category that included catheterization; teaching techniques and demonstrating them were combined in a single category; and the following categories were added to the list under nursing actions: (a) listens to fetal heart; (b) palpates abdomen, times contractions; (c) checks bladder, breasts, uterus, perineum; (d) touching, holding, cuddling, stroking; (e) temperature, pulse, respiratory, blood pressure; (f) checks supplies.

Results

The overall behavior of obstetric nurses in this sample, combining the high- and low-inference groups is as follows:

Verbal interactions. The most frequent category of verbal interaction was "explains, gives information," which occurred in nearly all the nurse-patient interactions observed. This was followed closely by "explores feelings" and "gives orders," both of which occurred in the majority of the interactions. "Sympathetic understanding, reassurance," and "verbalizes, explains actions to be taken" were next most frequent, with a sharp drop in frequency for all other verbal behaviors.

The observed differences in verbal behavior between obstetric and medical-surgical nurses obviously reflect the differences between the two nursing situations. Among medical-surgical nurses, the most frequent verbal behavior was "asks opening question," which usually initiated an interaction. In the medical-surgical unit, a patient feeling some distress typically called for a nurse, and in responding, the nurse's first step would be to find out why the patient called. In this setting, there is a wide range of reasons that might account for a patient's call, and the nurse's initial inquiry is clearly an important first step in most interactions. For the obstetric nurse, the range of likely problems is much more restricted, and contact with the patient does not depend nearly as often upon a patient's call. Thus, asking an opening question does not occur as often, because the nurse in most instances already knows the situation she will confront.

The following examples illustrate these differences in verbal behavior. Ms. Jones, a patient on the medical-surgical floor, was in her first postoperative day. Feeling some discomfort, she had switched on her call light. The nurse who responded to the signal had just come on duty. Although the nurse was aware that Ms. Jones had had a gall bladder operation, a wide range of reasons could have accounted for her call. Thus, the nurse's first step was an inquiry about what kind of help Ms. Jones required. The need to ask a direct question was typical of medical-surgical situations.

In contrast, let's consider Mrs. Planert, who was having her first baby. The nurse in attendance had been in and out of Mrs. Planert's room since her admission. The nurse knew Mrs. Planert's situation, and usually didn't depend on the patient's call to initiate an interaction. Thus, there was no need to ask an initial question.

Giving information and orders are high-frequency behaviors for both obstetric and medical-surgical nurses. However, exploring feelings and giving sympathetic understanding and reassurance were more characteristic of obstetrical nurses than of medical-surgical nurses. In Ms. Jones's case, she had a headache and the stitches were uncomfortable. The nurse checked the dressings and gave Ms. Jones several aspirin.

For Mrs. Planert, the obstetrical patient, the nurse was aware that the patient was in pain. When Mrs. Planert complained, the nurse remained at her side, reassuring her that everything was going along well. In contrast, the nurse did not ask Ms. Jones, the medical-surgical patient, if she was worried or upset, which may have been the cause of her headache.

Obstetric nurses explore their patient's feelings much more frequently than do medical-surgical nurses. Once again, this clearly reflects the difference in nursing situations; the obstetric nurse's actions depend to a certain extent on the patient's subjective report of her experiences, and thus, the nurse frequently seeks this information from the patient.

It should also be noted that sympathetic understanding and reassurance are expressed much more often by the obstetric nurse than by the medical-surgical nurse. This finding, too, reflects differences in the situations. In many instances, obstetric patients are clearly and obviously experiencing pain, and the nurse responds with understanding and reassurance. Among medical-surgical patients, the pain or psychological distress may not be so obvious, and the expression of sympathetic understanding is less frequently elicited.

The most frequent nursing actions were "straightens bedding, etc.," followed by "changes patient's position," "checks bladder, breasts, uterus, perineum," and "palpates abdomen, times contractions." These categories obviously reflect the particular demands of the obstetric nursing situation.

When we compare obstetric nurses with medical-surgical nurses, a number of differences are evident. For the obstetric nurses, several different nursing actions accounted for most of the interactions. In checking an obstetrical patient, there are set procedures which all the nurses followed. However, for the medical-surgical nurses, no single action was routinely followed. This finding undoubtedly reflects the heterogeneity of demands made upon medical-surgical nurses. The patients have varied illnesses and injuries, and a call for the nurse can come from a variety of patient needs.

Obstetric nurses more frequently engaged in straightening behaviors in comparison to medical-surgical nurses. It is difficult to be sure of what this finding means, but perhaps some of the obstetric nurses' straightening behaviors served as a tension-reducing mechanism for situations where there was a relatively high degree of tension.

Differences between High- and Low-Inference Obstetric Groups

Verbal interactions. There were differences between the high- and low-inference groups of obstetrical nurses in verbal interactions, nursing actions, and relations with patients. Nurses in the high-inference group more frequently expressed sympathetic understanding and reassurance to their patients. None of the other categories of verbal interaction showed significant differences between the two groups of nurses.

Let's consider Mrs. Planert's case again, as an example. When Ms. I., a high-inference nurse, routinely checked Mrs. Planert, she not only plumped pillows, changed a gown, and straightened the bedding, but held Mrs. Planert's hand during contractions. In one instance, she fixed Mrs. Planert's hair, saying, "You have a lovely head of hair, but I think you'll be more comfortable if I pull it back off your face."

While engaging in these touching behaviors, she offered reassurance and sympathy. "I know just how you feel. It won't be much longer. You are in very good shape. I know you won't have problems. Time seems to drag, but it really hasn't been all that long. Tomorrow at this time you'll be celebrating."

In contrast, Ms. B., a low-inference nurse, did not engage in the "extra touching" behaviors that characterized the high-inference nurse. Obviously, while working with Mrs. Planert, it was necessary for Ms. B. to touch her; however, all the touching was directly related to the examination. Although she did ask Mrs. Planert how she was feeling, her reassurance was brief, limited to such comments as, "You're doing fine, just fine. Everything is going along nicely"—generalized comments that tended to be impersonal.

Nursing actions and relations with patients. Both of the significant differences obtained in this study are in the direction expected and are congruent with the general trend of results obtained for medical-surgical nurses. Nevertheless, nurses in the high- and low-inference groups did not differ significantly in any of the other categories observed. Thus, for obstetric nurses, the expected relationship between beliefs and behavior is at best minimal, supported only by observations that high-inference nurses more often expressed sympathetic understanding and reassurance and touched their patients somewhat more frequently.

The results of this study suggest that the relationship between nurses' beliefs and their nursing behaviors is mitigated by the situation in which the nursing occurs. In an obstetric setting, perhaps the immediate situational demands are so compelling that the effects of a nurse's beliefs about patients' experiences are obscured. For example, during an obstetric patient's labor, a nurse's actions are likely to be determined primarily by her observation of physical signs that indicate the progress of the labor. It is generally assumed that the patient in labor will experience some pain, and while evidence of very severe distress will undoubtedly influence a nurse's behavior, relatively small differences in the amount of suffering inferred probably play a minor role in determining the obstetric nurse's actions. In obstetric nursing, then, situational factors rather than a particular nurse's beliefs may be the predominant influence on behavior.

Findings of Study Three: Pediatric Nurses

Having studied the relation between nurses' beliefs about suffering and their nursing behaviors among medical-surgical and obstetric nurses, a third study was undertaken to investigate the same relationship in still another setting. There were, of course, a number of possibilities that might have been selected, but a primary consideration at this stage of the research was to focus on a patient population that was clearly different from those found in a medical-surgical or obstetric unit. In the preceding studies, all the patients were adults, and this factor itself may have had some influence on the relation between nurses' beliefs and behaviors. Therefore, to investigate the same general problem with a distinctly different group of patients, nurses working in pediatric units were chosen as the focus of the third study in this series.

The design of this study repeated that of the preceding two studies, with the exception of the nature of the sample. As in the preceding studies, a nurse-observer accompanied each nurse in the sample and observed and recorded the nurse's interactions with patients. For the present study, one category, "adjusts language to patient," was added to the list of observed verbal interactions, and the three categories designed for the study of obstetric nursing ("listens to fetal heart," etc.) were omitted.

Results

By far the most frequent category of verbal interactions for all the pediatric nurses, including both high- and low-inference groups, was "explores feelings." "Explains, gives information" and "gives orders" were next highest in frequency, and just below this were "chats about condition," and "verbalizes, explains actions to be taken."

In general, these results suggest that the pediatric nurses in this sample talked with their patients much more than did the medical-surgical or obstetric nurses sampled in the preceding studies. Compare, for example, the results for pediatric and medical-surgical nurses in terms of two categories, "explores feelings" and "chats about condition." Both of these categories occurred in very few of the interactions observed among medical-surgical nurses and their patients. In contrast, both of these categories typically occurred for pediatric nurses. It would seem, therefore, that pediatric nurses, in comparison to medical-surgical nurses, spend a good deal more time chatting with their patients and exploring their patients' feelings.

The differences between pediatric and obstetric nurses are less striking than those between pediatric and medical-surgical nurses. For both pediatric and obstetric nurses, exploring patients' feelings occurred in many of the interactions observed. However, obstetric nurses much more frequently gave explanations and provided information to their patients. It would seem likely that this difference reflects differences both in the nursing tasks and the patient populations in obstetric and pediatric units.

The highest frequency categories of nursing actions for pediatric nurses in this sample were "adjusts I.V.," "T.P.R., blood pressure," "straightens bedding, etc.," and "touching, holding, cuddling, stroking." Thus, pediatric nurses most frequently engaged in the routines of nursing care (for example, T.P.R.), various straightening behaviors, and physical contact with their patients.

In general, pediatric nurses, on the average, performed more nursing actions than did medical-surgical nurses. The patterns of nursing actions for pediatric and obstetric nurses were similar in several respects, both groups showing high frequencies in adjusting patients' positions, various straightening behaviors, and physical contact with their patients. There were, of course, obvious differences with respect to categories of action specific to obstetric nursing (for example, "palpates abdomen, times contractions"). In addition, obstetric nurses engaged somewhat more often in teaching and demonstrating actions than did pediatric nurses.

Verbal interactions. High-inference pediatric nurses were significantly different from low-inference pediatric nurses in several categories. The high-inference nurses chatted with their patients considerably more often and expressed greater sympathetic understanding than did low-inference nurses. There were no differences between the two groups in any of the other categories.

Nursing actions. High-inference nurses more frequently changed their patients' positions and provided physical nurturing, while low-inference nurses more frequently engaged in straightening behaviors.

Relations with patients. Only one dimension showed a difference: nurses in the high-inference group were rated as somewhat warmer in emotional tone than were nurses in the low-inference group. None of the other dimensions revealed significant differences.

Results for pediatric nurses showed a number of differences in the expected direction. Pediatric nurses who tended to infer relatively high patient suffering also tended to chat with their patients and express sympathetic understanding and reassurance more often; they appeared to be more concerned with the comfortable positions of their patients, engaged more frequently in physical nurturing, and displayed straightening behaviors less often. Finally, they were rated as emotionally warmer in their overall interactions with patients. Thus, data obtained for the sample of pediatric nurses clearly support the proposition that nurses' beliefs about suffering are consistently and meaningfully related to their nursing behaviors.

Implications for Nursing

The results of the various studies strongly suggest that there is indeed a relationship between nurses' beliefs about suffering and their nursing behaviors. These findings add considerable weight to the results of previous investigations of nurses' inferences of suffering. In these earlier studies, we were primarily concerned with explicating nurses' implicit beliefs about suffering and determining those variables that influence inferences about the degree of pain and psychological distress experienced by patients. In the course of these investigations, a substantial number of findings were obtained, and much was learned about nurses' beliefs concerning suffering. However, until the present research, the concept of nurses' implicit beliefs about suffering was not empirically tied to actual nursing behavior. It seemed reasonable, of course, to assume that nurses' beliefs are related to their behaviors, but without clear-cut empirical evidence, this assumption remained untested. Thus, the results of the present investigation not only are interesting and valuable in terms of the specific issue studied, but they also validate the usefulness of our earlier research. By virtue of the present findings, the concept of nurses' implicit beliefs about suffering moves from an interesting theoretical construct to a variable that is directly and empirically tied to actual nursing practice.

Although nurses' beliefs and behaviors are generally related, the specific nature of the relationship depends upon the particular setting considered. In the three studies reported in this series, there was no single category of either verbal interaction or nursing action and no single dimension of relations with patients that revealed significant differences for nurses in all three settings. Medical-surgical nurses who tended to infer relatively high suffering in patients also tended to explain their actions to patients more frequently and to dismiss less frequently their patients' concerns. But among obstetric nurses, nurses in both high- and low-inference groups frequently explained their actions to patients and rarely dismissed their patients' concerns. Similarly, pediatric nurses who tended to infer relatively high suffering also tended to express sympathetic understanding more frequently and to chat about the patients' condition. But among medical-surgical nurses, neither high- nor low-inference nurses devoted much time to chatting with patients about their conditions and did not very frequently express sympathetic understanding and reassurance. Thus, we can conclude that the setting in which nurses work has a very important impact on the ways in which their beliefs are reflected in their behaviors.

Support for this proposition derives from a comparison of results for obstetric and medical-surgical nurses. In the medical-surgical setting, significant differences were obtained for three categories of verbal interactions, two categories of nursing actions, and three dimensions dealing with the nurses' relations with patients. In the obstetric setting, however, significant differences were obtained for only two categories of verbal interactions, only one category of nursing actions, and for none of the dimensions dealing with relations with patients. For the medical-surgical nurses, we can conclude that there is apparently a good deal of opportunity for beliefs to be expressed in behaviors. There is often enough leeway in the medical-surgical unit to permit a range of adequate nursing behaviors. For the obstetric nurses, however, the immediate demands of the situation are likely to be much more restrictive on behavior.

Obstetric nurses cannot remain physically distant from the patients; they must inquire about the patients' feelings in order to function appropriately; when patients experience pain, the evidence of this pain is obvious and the nurses cannot readily or reasonably dismiss the patients' concern. Furthermore, the obstetric nurses' actions are likely to be determined largely by the patients' physical condition, and in comparison to the medical-surgical nurses, the obstetric nurses have a relatively restricted range of tasks to perform. Situational factors probably exert a greater influence on obstetric nurses' behavior, and as a result, the relation between beliefs and behaviors is more tenuous than that for medical-surgical nurses.

Further evidence in support of the differential effects of various situations derives from a consideration of the overall behavior of the combined groups of nurses in each of the three settings. Consider, for example, the pediatric nurses, in contrast to the medical-surgical nurses. The pediatric nurses talked much more with the children who were their patients. They spent a good deal of time chatting with the children about their condition, exploring the children's feelings, and offering sympathetic understanding and reassurance. In contrast, the medical-surgical nurses engaged in these kinds of verbal interactions much less often. There is no evidence to support the assumption that medical-surgical nurses are any less sensitive to or concerned about their patients than are the pediatric nurses, and there is no significant difference in their beliefs about suffering. It would seem most reasonable, therefore, to interpret the observed differences in nursing behaviors as a function of differences in the situations in which pediatric and medical-surgical nurses work. Informal observations during the course of this research suggested that pediatric nurses often have much more opportunity to talk with their patients, and informal chatting with the children in their unit is more likely to be viewed as an intrinsic part of pediatric nursing care. Medical-surgical nurses, on the other hand, appeared to have less opportunity for informal conversation with patients and seemed less likely to view such conversation as a significant part of their nursing responsibilities.

From a theoretical point of view, the results of this series of studies tend to support an interpretation of low inferences of suffering as a reflection, in part, of a defensive or protective mechanism used by the nurse. This mechanism is similar to Harry Stack Sullivan's concept of selective inattention as a means of dealing with anxiety. According to Sullivan, a commonly used technique for reducing anxiety is a selective lack of attention to the source of the threat. In colloquial terms, if you don't pay attention to the threat, you won't feel so anxious, and maybe it will go away.

For some nurses, patients' suffering may be a source of threat that elicits anxiety. Forced to deal on a day-to-day basis with people who are in pain and experiencing psychological distress, and confronted by the fact that on some occasions the nurses cannot significantly relieve the patients' suffering, a selective lack of attention to this suffering may be a very effective way for the nurses to maintain their own psychological integrity. Believing that patients do not suffer a great deal of pain or psychological distress is a form of selective inattention, and our measure of low inferences of suffering may reflect, in part, this mechanism. Just as the low-inference nurses' belief systems reflect this mechanism, so too do their nursing behaviors reflect a tendency to be selectively inattentive to the experiences of the patients. Thus, low-inference nurses may appear to act insensitively, although this behavior may in fact be a consequence of their sensitivity to the patients' suffering and the anxiety that this suffering elicits in the nurses.

To a certain extent, most people who work closely with those who are suffering probably use one form or another of selective inattention. It is a psychological mechanism commonly used in everyday life to deal with anxiety-inducing situations, and there is no reason to believe that nurses are exempt from using this mechanism. A problem in nursing care arises, however, when this mechanism takes an extreme form. As indicated by this research, low inferences of suffering are associated with nursing behaviors that maintain psychological distance between nurses and patients. Nurses that are psychologically distant are less likely to take the patients' feelings into account, and thus, they are probably less effective in relieving the patients' distress.

The problem for nursing, then, is to devise means of guarding against overreactions to patient suffering that lead to psychologically protective mechanisms that interfere with effective nursing care.

Although it is obviously very important for nurses to be in touch with their patients' feelings, overreactions to patients' suffering can interfere with nurses' functioning. Thus, nurses must learn to be sensitive to their patients' feelings, but at the same time maintain their professional role in providing care. It is this subtle and complex balance of interpersonal sensitivity and professional self-control that characterizes the truly effective nurse.

9

The Empathic Nurses

In the course of our research, we had a chance to observe a large number of nurses who clearly provided very efficient and effective care for their patients. Among these excellent nurses, however, a relatively small group seemed to stand out from the rest. These were the nurses who were especially sensitive to their patients' feelings, took extra care and time in their relationships with patients, and seemed to provide an "extra dimension" of nursing care. In the more technical aspects of nursing, their behavior was not very different from other excellent nurses we observed. They were efficient, obviously knowledgeable, and highly skilled. But their nursing was comprised of something more than efficiency, knowledge, and technical skills.

From time to time, we took the opportunity to talk with these nurses, and occasionally, to accompany them as they worked. Gradually, we came to recognize that the special quality characteristic of these nurses was a highly refined empathic response to their patients. They seemed to be very much "in touch" with their patients' experiences, particularly with regard to their patients' pain and psychological distress. We called this group "the empathic nurses."

Obviously, almost all the nurses we have studied in our research have the capacity to empathize with the experiences of their patients. Thus, the empathic nurse did not have some unique quality that was not shared with other nurses. It seemed to be a matter of degree. Those we came to call the empathic nurses displayed a level of sensitivity that was, at least statistically, most unusual.

As a result of these informal observations, we decided to study the unusually empathic nurse somewhat more systematically. The present study represents only a small first step in this direction. It was highly exploratory and was aimed only at discovering some possible further research. The results, therefore, must not be viewed as a basis for firm conclusions, but rather, as suggestions that may lead to further study.

Selecting the Empathic Nurses

From the total group of medical-surgical, pediatric, and obstetric nurses observed in the three studies dealing with inferences of suffering and nursing behaviors (Chapter 8), ten nurses were selected on the basis of the following criteria: (1) high scores on the *Standard Measure of Inferences of Suffering;* (2) high scores on the categories of observed behaviors that indicated active concern with the patient's feelings. These included, for example, exploring patients' feelings, expressing sympathetic understanding, and various nurturing actions. Thus, the ten empathic nurses we studied were selected on the basis of both test results indicating sensitivity to patients' suffering and observations of actual nursing behaviors reflecting active concern for patients' feelings.

The nurses in the sample ranged in age from 22 to 55 years. Four were working on medical-surgical floors; three were in pediatrics; three were in obstetrics. The group came from strikingly different ethnic backgrounds, for example, black American, Russian-Polish, Jewish, Italian, Irish, Puerto Rican, West Indies, Maltese, German, and Caribbean.

The Interview

Each of the ten empathic nurses was interviewed individually. These interviews were relatively informal and open-ended. The participants were told that we were interested in learning something about their backgrounds and their views of nursing, and after the initial question about why the nurse had entered nursing, the interviewer merely reflected what the nurse said or followed up any leads in the nurse's comments by open-ended questions, such as, "Tell me more about that," or "Could you explain that more fully."

Findings

The results of these interviews are summarized in terms of the major themes that emerged from the nurses' comments. In each case, the theme was mentioned independently by at least seven of the ten nurses, and in some instances was discussed by all ten nurses. Thus, the findings reported here represent more or less common themes mentioned by the ten nurses who were interviewed.

Decision to Become a Nurse

In considering their motivation to enter nursing, there was no single motive or pattern of motivation that characterized this group. The reasons underlying their decisions to become nurses included a variety of factors, such as a search for a more meaningful life, a sense of responsibility to others, family encouragement, and chance.

"My mother had to take care of the family by herself. My father died when I was nine. Even though we had very little ourselves, my mother always put aside some food for someone who might be hungry. She was always helping friends and relatives. I guess it was kind of natural that when I was ready to choose a career I would decide on one that let me play this role."

"I come from a deeply religious family. They all had a tremendous responsibility to help others. Family duties and helping people were part of my upbringing. Several aunts were nurses, and it was always understood in the family that I would follow them to England and train. The idea that nursing meant working with sick people, dealing with death and dying, never bothered me. I come from a culture where death is not feared. My mother had her clothes all ready for her burial even though she wasn't ill. Us kids knew about death. Death was part of our life. We even had prayers praying for death in our church."

"My parents wanted me to go to nursing school so I'd have a profession. They helped me financially. When I graduated, it meant a lot to them as well as to me. When I got my degree, I had a great sense of accomplishment, and the family—everyone—came to a huge party."

"I was brought up in a rural area. My great grandmother was a nurse-midwife. As a kid, I often went with her to watch. I saw how much she meant to the women and how big a role she played in the lives of people. I might not have been aware of it at the time, but all this influenced my decision to become a nurse. I wanted to have the same kind of importance and respect. I knew I could achieve this with a career in nursing."

"We were very poor. My family came to the states from Puerto Rico. My father got ill; my mother stayed home to take care of the kids. We were on welfare. Neither of my parents had much education. My father quit school in the fifth grade; my mother only went to the second grade. It was her dream that her children would have an education. My twin sister and I played nurse when we were small. My mother bought us nurses' kits. When we were fourteen, we became volunteers at a hospital, and were always called back because we were so reliable. Going to nursing school, for both me and my sister, was a natural step, with all our experience as teenagers."

"I went into nursing more by chance than anything else. I was the youngest of a large family. None of the others had gone on to school. I was the only one who expressed a desire. My parents had a real struggle getting together the $100 tuition. It meant a big sacrifice at the time. I really didn't know what nursing was all about. I wanted to go on to school, and my two best friends had enrolled in nursing school. I just followed them."

"I started as a 'psych' major in college. It was dull for me. It wasn't satisfying. I was drifting that year. About the middle of the term, I happened to go to a career conference and talked with this dynamic, elderly woman. She struck me as very real. She was warm, wholesome, and I mean that in a positive way. I was impressed with her scholarship. She made sense, and I went back to the dorm to think about what she had said. A couple of weeks later, I went back to see her and told her I had decided to switch to nursing."

"I've always loved kids and I started out in school wanting to be a primary school teacher. I used to babysit a lot and I worked as a camp counselor. After I started practice teaching in a kindergarten I realized it wasn't for me. I didn't seem to be doing anything meaningful. I was really trying to find myself. I remembered a nurse who worked for a pediatrician I had gone to as a child and I thought about it for awhile and realized that if I wanted to work with children in a meaningful way that I would become a nurse."

"I remembered when I was a kid I was sick and I had a nurse who was horrible. I know it sounds funny but the memory of her stuck with me and I made up my mind to go to nursing school and become the kind of nurse who cared."

"I was a loner as a kid. I was interested in people but stayed by myself. I wanted to become an undertaker. I was quite serious about this. I thought that I could help people when they needed it most—families who had a death. I guess I thought more about death than most kids. When I was 12, my brother who was 8 was killed by a hit-and-run driver. My dad took it badly. Anyhow, I gave up the undertaker idea. I was married, had a child, divorced. For about ten years I supported myself and my child working on the stock exchange. I made good money, and I had a terrific career ahead of me. One day out of the blue I asked myself what is life all about? I felt I had to do something more meaningful with my life than work with columns of figures. I went back to school at night. And then the idea of becoming a nurse to help people crossed my mind. I made my decision and went into training."

Commitment to Nursing

Although the nurses in this group entered the field for a variety of reasons, once they became nurses, they were strongly committed to nursing. For them nursing was much more than the usual job; it was a central source of satisfaction, pride, and meaningfulness in their lives.

"When I go to work, I feel good. I like what I do. I count in other people's lives, and I never forget that for one minute. I feel very committed to nursing. Sure there are irritations, but every job has problems."

"Around the hospital, they call me 'Little Florence Nightingale.' I don't mind being teased. There's a lot of truth in what they call me. I have never lost sight of the fact that this is my life, my career. I'm not going to compromise myself or get embarrassed about being dedicated."

"When I can't get into work, I feel guilty. Nursing isn't something you can do one day and then take off the rest of the week. People count on me. I don't feel I have the right to let them down. I try to get into work no matter what."

"I love my work. I know that sounds corny but when I'm at work I feel like I'm in a 'bubble.' Nothing in the outside world comes between me and my job—my daughter, my husband, my family."

"There never has been a single day when I haven't wanted to go to work. It's as simple as that."

"Nursing isn't a nine-to-five job. Sometimes it's more. I don't feel that it is a job, because I get a sense of fulfillment about my days. Some of the girls think about just getting through seven or eight hours, and then they can do something they enjoy. I don't feel like that. I enjoy what I'm doing."

The one person who did not share this sense of commitment had been a professional nurse for less than a year. Her feelings about work were mixed. On the one hand, she enjoyed what she was doing, but the pleasure was tempered by the day-to-day frustrations she encountered. "It might be where I'm working, I'm not sure. Lots of things bother me, like having to spend so much time with paperwork—far more than the time I can spend with patients."

Nursing Education

Almost without exception, the group described its years in training as rigorous, demanding, and highly structured. Occasionally, they resented the demands and the discipline, but in retrospect, they talked about their experiences in nursing school with a great sense of pride. Having succeeded under the stressful and demanding conditions of their various nursing schools, they felt they could handle just about any challenge they met in their nursing career. Thus, their educational experiences were a significant source of professional confidence.

"My school was very demanding. I can't remember one instructor who didn't know what she was doing. They were the most professional people I've ever met. The school never 'slacked' off. There wasn't a moment we weren't 'hit' with the philosophy that if something was worth doing, it was worth doing well."

"There was no leeway given to the student who was careless or sloppy. If a girl remained that way, she was dismissed. We had to conform to standards. I remember being constantly evaluated. There wasn't an aspect where we weren't judged—our manners, dress, behavior. There were no exceptions. I recall the demanding aspects of training; at the time I got angry. Some girls couldn't take it and left. Now I'm glad I stuck it out. I learned confidence. I think the nurses who aren't satisfied are the least competent."

"I went to a school run by the Dominican Fathers. The sisters were Sisters of Charity. They had very high demands. Our skirts had to be two inches below the knees or we were reprimanded. They actually measured if there was a question. We weren't allowed to wear jewelry, makeup. The external controls imposed on the students helped us to gain internal discipline. We weren't allowed to let off steam. We had to have external controls, no matter what we felt inside. I know that the way I act toward patients is because of my training. The school's philosophy was that patients must be treated with respect at all times. We were told over and over again that patients were individuals and must be reacted to with consideration. Patient needs were first and foremost."

"My school was concerned with every part of our lives. Where I'm working, students will come on the floor having had only a cup of coffee and a cigarette at breakfast. I couldn't imagine anything like this happening to me as a student. Our matron (an English school) always gave us lectures about how we must start the day off with a proper breakfast. This is just an example of how everything that went on with students was a concern of the faculty. I'm sure that I gained considerable strength and discipline for having come up through a system that had very high standards of deportment and training.''

"My school was impossibly strict when compared to schools nowadays. I loved every minute of it. Maybe it was easier for me to accept than it was for some of the other girls. I had been brought up in a strict home where you had to obey your elders or else! The teachers at school actually were easier than my own family in some ways. We were checked constantly. We had to know our patients; we had to know what was going on; we couldn't get away with laziness, not caring, not knowing. If we didn't know something, it was up to us to find out.''

"My biggest memory of nursing school was being a lowly probie and holding my breath when the director of the school walked by. We were watched, kept in check. For the first six months, we couldn't make a move without someone breathing over our shoulder. After the first six months, we were given responsibilities. There was a dramatic shift and we were aware of the responsibility being given to us and the independence. I'm grateful for that kind of rigorous training I had. I learned confidence.''

Only one woman reported attending a boring, mechanical baccalaureate program. She had found only one faculty member empathic to students' needs. "If it hadn't been for this one woman, I probably would have left training. She was warm, sensitive, and loving. I can't ever remember her cutting a student down or cutting the amount of time she spent with us. But school wasn't very exciting. It was something to get through with as quickly as possible.''

Role Models

Role models encountered during training or early in practice exercised an enormous influence on the majority of these nurses. In describing these models, the nurses mentioned characteristics such as self-discipline, calmness, confidence, poise, and commitment. But regardless of the various characteristics mentioned, for most of these nurses, there was someone in their backgrounds whom they viewed as an ideal nurse and whom they tried to emulate.

"I vividly remember two people who made a big impression on me. I wanted to be like them, though at the time it seemed impossible. Still in all, it didn't keep me from trying. One was the school director. It's been over thirty years since I was a student and I can still picture her, slim, blonde, always dignified and poised. She was so confident and assured. Sort of an immaculate kind of person, if you know what I mean. She had a great way with the students. They all loved her."

"Mac was a small, bustling Scotch woman. I don't know what we would have done without Mac. She backed us up. Her philosophy was that we could do anything if we tried. All of us wanted very much to please Mac, not to let her down. Other staff members yelled, criticized us publicly—never Mac. She never raised her voice, and if she had anything to say to us, she made sure she talked privately. Mac was devoted to nursing, and had such a 'jolly' attitude. I've never met anyone in all my experience who could make patients and staff feel so reassured."

"I worked with Shirley my first year out of school. I used to watch her and hope that I would become like her. She could go from bed to bed, never losing her calmness, never getting uptight, but doing things constantly to make patients happy."

"The greatest impression made on me was a supervisor. I used to marvel at the way she could take a staff member who had a problem and needed to talk and turn what could be an awful situation into a positive one. Her strength was unbelievable. She kept everyone going—helpful to the patients and everyone on the staff."

"I always think about one nurse when things get tough and I've had it for the day. She was calm, dignified. I thought how great it was the way she could be such a ramrod of strength. She was dedicated. I wanted very much to win her approval and tried to be like her. I think I still do. I know I never lived up to her expectations at the time, and I'm not the sort of person who never breaks, but I keep trying. She made me feel so good about myself. Never did she let on that I had failed or did something wrong. She was the same way with everyone."

Although the vast majority of the group had been influenced through positive encounters with outstanding nurses, one woman stressed the impact "bad nurses" had on her performance. For this individual, observations of what she termed "poor nursing" made the greatest impression.

"What I mean is that when I worked with a nurse who was hostile and mean to patients, I'd say to myself, 'I'm never going to be like that, no matter what.' I've worked with staff who resented every minute on the floor. That bothered me. Again, I'd think to myself, 'If that day comes, I'm going to leave nursing.' It's not a matter of age, I've found out. I've met older nurses who are warm, kind, take the time to help younger nurses, who are great with patients. I've watched young nurses behave the same way. The hard, angry ones can be old or young. It doesn't matter. I'm convinced it's the individual and not the age or anything else that makes a difference."

Self-Esteem

Perhaps the most striking and consistent characteristic shared by all of these nurses was their professional self-esteem. They knew they were good nurses and conveyed their self-evaluation, not with any sense of bragging or boasting, but with quiet, secure confidence.

"Nursing to me is a total kind of thing, not something I do only for money. Sure, I like to get paid for what I do, but I'm a nurse in uniform or out of uniform. What I am trying to say is that basically, I respect the kind of person I am. I don't put on a uniform like a mask and turn on caring, or whatever. I am myself at work or out of work, and this makes a huge difference in how I feel about my job and myself. I know a lot of people can't wait until the end of the day and they can 'become themselves.' I am myself at work—the same kind of person when I'm out with friends or at home."

"I happen to believe in myself and what I do. I know I have one fault that drives some people wild. I am a perfectionist. It doesn't bother me, though, because I'm not going to compromise my professional standards or my own standards for anyone or anything."

"I feel sure of myself and what I do. Perhaps this is because I've come up the hard way. Maybe I would be different if I had had a middle-class background. I don't know. I've pulled myself up from the bottom and I know what it's like to come from a family on welfare and parents who had no education. I've been on the other side, and I've accomplished a great deal. I respect what I've done. I don't mean I have to go around convincing people I'm somebody. I'm confident. This doesn't mean I still don't have a lot to learn."

"I know where I'm going and what I'm doing. I never feel hopeless or helpless. There are plenty of times I don't know what to do or have doubts, but I'm never at a total loss."

Respect from Colleagues

In addition to their self-esteem, these nurses were also secure in their sense of being respected by others. Thus, each nurse's self-concept as an effective nurse was reinforced by the evaluations of others with whom she worked.

"In all the years I've worked, I've never felt that doctors didn't respect what I do. Maybe it's the group I work with. I am free to make decisions. The doctors on the staff thank me. Many times they'll tell me to use my judgment, 'We trust you.' When I have to telephone a doctor and tell him to come, he responds immediately. He knows I wouldn't call unless it was absolutely necessary. I'm talking about the staff doctors. I know what I'm saying doesn't hold up always with some of the others who use our hospital facilities."

"I'm not the kind of person who sits back and takes what is handed out from other people without a word. If I'm right, I'll stand up for my rights. No one can stand in my way. Doctors and other nurses know the way I am and they respect me. I treat them with respect, and I've never failed to be treated in the same way."

"I'm a fighter. If I'm right, I'll hold to my opinion. That bothers some people. But I do listen. If I'm proven wrong, I'm the first one to admit my error. I think because of the way I am, my co-workers and the doctors respect me. No one respects a person who lets herself be walked over. I'll have doctors ask my opinion. It's very important for me to have my judgments respected."

"I know a lot of nurses complain about doctors not respecting them. I think I do have the respect of my co-workers. The fault isn't so much with the doctors, I think, as it is with the system. In my hospital, we never have group discussions about patients. There are no chances to get together to discuss patients. The hospital respects the doctors, but forgets about nurses' needs. I think that if we had a chance to sit down together as a group to review cases, there would be a huge difference in the kind of respect doctors had for nurses, and the other way around."

"Respect from doctors depends on the doctor. But then that's true with the other nurses. I think I'm respected, even though I disagree a lot with other people. I feel pretty confident and sometimes people resent this, though they have to respect me for holding to my opinions when I'm right and they know I'm right."

"My supervisor disturbs me the way she behaves towards the doctors. She shakes when they come around. I don't think they respect her more because she fawns all over them. I don't want to behave like that. I am not defensive. I know my job; I respect my colleagues and I want to be treated the same way. I think because I am sure of myself and I am not apologetic or submissive, I'm respected more."

Caring for Others

Caring for others was unquestionably the most important source of professional satisfaction reported by these nurses. They emphasized the intrinsic reward they experienced in helping another person, as well as the appreciation expressed by others.

"My satisfactions in nursing come from working with people who are sick and seeing them get better and ready to go home. I like the feeling of being appreciated by the patients, that I helped make this possible. When they show they trust me and respect me, I feel good about myself and my work."

"The most rewarding part of nursing is patient contact. I enjoy being looked up to by the patients. I enjoy relating to them in a personal sort of way. My greatest satisfactions come when patients welcome me. They feel I understand them. I like being thought of as someone special. I know this is a fact, because I get feedback. There is laughter, conversation. Then many times, others on the staff will tell me that so-and-so was asking for the nurse with the long braid. I get a glow of satisfaction when I hear this.''

"I get a sense of fulfillment about my days. The rewards for me come when I help someone. I know when patients express appreciation—a small gift, a box of candy, and there's nothing wrong with these things—I have a sense of achievement, well-being.''

"I think there is nothing greater than a feeling of having helped someone. I think being empathic as a nurse is so important. There is a line between you and the patient, but reaching out and knowing you have succeeded is a good feeling.''

"I enjoy being liked and needed. The satisfaction I get comes from my patients and this is very important for me. When I see a patient ready for discharge, standing up straight, getting ready to leave the hospital and feeling good, I share the feeling.''

Relating to Patients

Throughout the interviews, the nurse's relationship with the patient was repeatedly emphasized as the core of nursing. This central concept was expressed in a variety of ways, but in one way or another, all the nurses underscored the crucial importance of how they related to patients.

Some of the nurses talked about the time they devoted to their relationships with patients.

"It gripes me to hear nurses talk about not having enough time to do the kind of job they want to. It's just an excuse. There's always enough time. Somehow you can find the time if you really care.''

"My biggest problem with patients is getting overwhelmed. My supervisor is always after me for being slow. I find I want to spend time with patients. I do what is necessary for each one and then go on to the next step. My supervisor doesn't see it this way. She is always hurrying everyone. Even though I get my work done, she says I'm slow. I really don't want to change. Caring for patients is what nursing is all about.''

"I think it's nonsense that nurses don't have enough time to be kind or caring. Even on the busiest days, you can be sympathetic. When I'm rushed and can't take time, I go back later in the day. No one would stop any nurse from going back to a patient when the nurse had more time. I think our profession would do itself a great service if we stopped blaming the clock for our behavior. It doesn't help the nurse or the patients to use time as a reason for the way we might behave."

A number of the nurses talked about the ways in which they related to especially difficult patients.

"When patients are hostile, I tell myself they're not rational. It makes me angry when nurses reject patients they say are hostile or demanding. I have never yet failed to believe that a call is an honest call for help. It might not seem like that sometimes, because of the kind of request or question the patient has. But there's a reason. It could be they're upset and need a little attention. I think I'm like a lot of nurses and I have problems handling psychological distress. It's a lot easier to handle the physical complaints. And I know that a call for psychological help is as real as anything else. One of my friends who is a nurse lost a baby. Everyone stayed away, saying they didn't know what to say to her. I went in and we talked. She got a chance to tell someone how awful she felt. All she needed was someone to listen to her."

"I never really become upset with hostile or demanding patients. It always flashes through my mind that the patient isn't accountable for what she might be saying or doing. In another situation, that patient could be a completely different person. I think I can cope with patient aggression because I never take it personally. Some nurses do, and that's a mistake."

"Hospital patients never throw me. I know they are displacing their anger at themselves onto me. I always tell myself, when I walk into a new patient's room and they are angry with me, how could it really be me when they don't even know me. I know the patient is angry at being in the hospital. I never show anger in return."

Many of the nurses in this group emphasized their sense of respect and caring for patients.

"I respect my patients. I respect them and I want to be respected. I think my respect for patients comes from my training. I was taught that we always had time to put ourselves in the other person's place. I find many times thinking this could be my sister, my father, my mother. How would I want them treated?''

"I have a child, and I believe that if I behave in a caring way toward my patients, toward everybody, my child will receive rewards. This is part of my culture to think like this. I think that people from the Islands are more humanistic. American nurses seem much less sympathetic. They're caught up in the technical part of nursing and seem to forget people are in those beds and not machines.''

"I respect every patient where I work. I know what it feels like to sit on a bench in an out-patient clinic. I sat there many times with my mother or father. I know how awful we felt when some nurse was rude to my mother and I knew she was sick. I'll never behave that way. I know what it is like to be on the other side.''

"In nursing school and at work, we're always being told to distance ourselves from our patients. I don't agree. I don't think I could be a good nurse and not care. It's impossible to disassociate yourself from patients. I think of the way I behave as controlled disassociation. I have to care, and yet I have to have control of my empathy or I can't do a good job.''

"No matter what a patient says or does, I keep trying and caring. It never fails to win a patient over. When I go into someone who is very sick and that person is rude or unpleasant, I look at the patient and ask myself how I would feel if that were me in that bed. How would I behave? Some patients are stoic and cheerful. Most people, though, give in more to themselves when the situation is bad enough. When I think about how I would behave if it were me, I can't possibly do anything that would be hurtful.''

Teaching

Although caring for others was the primary source of professional satisfaction, a second area mentioned by several nurses was teaching. Thus, they viewed as an important part of caring for others the process of teaching others to care for themselves.

"Teaching is a part of nursing that is very important to me. I enjoy teaching. It's not just enough for a nurse to go into a patient and do the necessary things. It's just as important to teach the patients to care for themselves."

"I think patient teaching is the most important part of my work. I know that I enjoy this role very much. I could do with a lot less paperwork. We write instead of teach. I think many nurses hold back, don't spend enough time instructing their patients. I know that I feel an obligation to my patients to explain procedures, to talk with them about what I am doing instead of engaging in a lot of idle chit-chat. Patients appreciate being taught."

Personal Lives

Life outside of nursing was described as very satisfying. They experienced normal ups and downs, but in general, they expressed a sense of enjoyment in their friends, families, and activities outside the hospital.

"Nursing takes a big chunk of time in my life. I never resent it. I think a lot has to do with my family and friends. I'll meet someone and they find out I'm a nurse and they're impressed. My family thinks what I'm doing is the greatest. I guess I'm lucky this way. Lots of my friends have jobs they hate; they feel they aren't doing anything meaningful. One of my old high school friends keeps telling me she wished she had gone to nursing school instead of straight college. She ended up as a super secretary and can't wait to get out of the office."

"My husband is very proud of me. He's always telling people he's married to a nurse. There's never been a time when he hasn't pitched in with the housework or taking care of the kids because I've been too tired. The extra income is important, but that's not all there is to it. I know he respects my being a professional."

"I think part of why I enjoy what I'm doing is because it's not my whole life. I mean if all I had was nursing, I don't think I'd be happy. It gets kind of depressing at times. But I have a good social life. I'm in no rush to get married; I have a steady boyfriend. We probably will end up getting married next year. But now both of us like the freedom."

"It makes a big difference if you have other people in your life besides nurses and people from the hospital. I know that I count a lot on my family and friends. I think I'd be different if after work I went back to an empty house."

Discussion

In many respects, the nurses we talked to in this study were very different from one another. They came from widely different backgrounds, entered nursing for a variety of reasons, worked in a diversity of hospital settings, and their styles of personal life varied greatly. There were several interrelated themes that characterized their comments about nursing. These themes might be viewed in terms of commitment, confidence, and caring.

Commitment

Having entered nursing for many different reasons, once they became nurses, there was no question about their dedication and commitment to nursing. In our conversations with them, they were certainly not unrealistically idealistic or at all concerned with trying to impress us with their altruistic motivations. If anything, we would characterize them as down-to-earth, practical-minded professionals. But it was clear, nevertheless, that nursing for them meant much more than a mere job. It is difficult to capture the essense of all their comments; each of them was too much of an individual to fit into a single mold. Perhaps the closest we can come is to say that, from their different perspectives, they viewed nursing as a calling, rather than as just another job. In saying that they viewed nursing as a calling, we do not mean to suggest any religious implications; however, for this group, nursing was a profoundly meaningful part of their lives. It was not the only source of meaning; their interests and activities outside nursing were both generally varied and satisfying. But the values derived from nursing were extraordinarily important to them.

On the basis of our interviews, we cannot determine how this sense of personal and professional commitment developed. From their reports, it did not seem that this commitment was present for most of them when they entered nursing. Rather, it developed during their training and later experiences as nurses. There does not appear to be one way of achieving this commitment. Each nurse in her own unique way discovered the meaningfulness of nursing for herself, and as a result of this gradual process of discovery, became increasingly, committed to nursing as a central aspect of her life.

Confidence

In addition to a sense of commitment, each of these nurses clearly expressed confidence in herself as an effective nurse. Thus, they not only enjoyed what they were doing, but they also knew that they were doing it well. This self-esteem was reinforced both by appreciation from their patients and respect from their colleagues.

Frankly, their comments about the demanding and structured nature of their nursing education at first surprised us. We had not anticipated this finding, though it became less and less surprising as each successive nurse in the course of our interviews independently described the rigor of her training. We do not believe that the rigor of training in and of itself made these nurses especially empathic. Their training, however, contributed to their self-esteem and confidence, which permitted them to deal with the stresses of patient care without feeling threatened. They expressed a good deal of pride in the fact that they had successfully passed a very difficult course of training and felt that in this training, they had acquired the personal and professional skills necessary to function effectively, regardless of the particular problems they encountered in their nursing careers.

Caring

There was never any question about the purely technical competence of the nurses we talked to; in fact, part of their confidence was based on their secure knowledge of the more technical aspects of nursing care. But in discussing their views of nursing care, they went far beyond technical competence. They emphasized their own need to care for others and the importance of their relationships with patients. They took the time to care, were not unduly disturbed by very difficult patients, and respected the people with whom they worked.

Of the many factors that contributed to the development of this general attitude toward patient care, the nurses in this group focused particularly on the influence of role models early in their nursing careers. They all had had an opportunity to observe another nurse, usually a person in a senior position, who represented for them an ideal nurse, and the theme of caring was an important part of this ideal.

The Empathic Nurses

There is no simple way of describing or explaining the personal and professional development of an especially empathic nurse. It is much too complex a problem to be dealt with adequately in one very limited investigation. Nevertheless, the three interrelated themes of commitment, confidence, and caring would seem worth considering in further study. In this preliminary research, we feel that we have only scratched the surface of a very important problem, and the questions raised by this pilot investigation are far more significant than any tentative conclusions we might suggest. For example, how can nursing education foster and enhance a student's sense of commitment to nursing? Is a very demanding, highly structured, and rigorous course of training consistently related to the development of a sense of commitment and confidence, as is suggested by the information these nurses offered? How can the conditions of nursing practice be designed to reinforce nurses' self-esteem and confidence? What are the factors in current practice that work against the development of professional self-esteem? How can nursing schools achieve an appropriate balance between emphasizing high-level technical competence and recognizing the importance of interpersonal processes in nursing? Can we identify potentially important role models, and how can the impact of these role models be enhanced?

These are only a few of the questions raised by this preliminary study, and it is quite obvious that our research has resulted in many more questions being raised than answers even tentatively given. Addressing these questions in further research, however, may provide information on which to base a systematic foundation for future advances in the education of nurses and the practice of nursing.

10

The Effects of Education on Student Nurses' Inferences of Physical Pain and Psychological Distress

"It was awful those first weeks," Carol, a freshman nursing student, told us. After graduating from high school, she had worked in a day-care center and a nursing home for a year before entering a diploma program. "I thought I knew something about sick people. I had worked in the nursing home, and a lot of the older people were sick. I wasn't upset by what I saw. In fact, working in the home was what made me want to become a nurse. It was a lot different when I started school. I was in for a big shock. I can remember an instructor taking us on a hospital tour. We watched a nurse change a dressing. The man was in terrible pain. He yelled at the nurse. There was all this blood. I thought I was going to faint. I wondered how I could last in training. My stomach was turning over. The nurses we saw were so 'cool.' After class we were supposed to have lunch. I won't tell you what happened to me."

Carol's report about her feelings of being upset at first encounters with patient pain in school was not unique. As part of our study, we investigated students' beliefs about suffering and how these beliefs changed over the course of their education. Other freshman students reported experiences similar to Carol's.

June, an 18-year-old, stated, "Nothing in my life really prepared me for the reality. I remember when my brother broke his leg and he

was in pain. I was in the hospital for an operation, and I was pretty uncomfortable. I thought I had a good idea of what pain was like. It
wasn't the case. I think it's because it's different when you're a student
and see so many people all at once. Before school, you only know a few
cases—someone in your family, maybe, or yourself. In school now, I
see case after case. It's very hard in the beginning.''

Many first-year nursing students share the feelings expressed by
these two girls. Obviously there are exceptions; however, for the majority, the reality of confronting, day after day, situations involving patient suffering is a new experience. The effect on attitudes is inevitable.

Not only are freshmen students influenced by reality, they are
also affected by academic studies. Textbooks, lectures, filmstrips, ex-
pose them to more academically oriented considerations of suffering
that accompany illness. Thus, from the very start of training, student
attitudes and beliefs are shaped by academic as well as clinical
involvement.

The purpose of our research was to consider these effects on
students' beliefs about suffering. The overall question raised was
whether attitudes toward patient suffering change with increasing
clinical exposure and formal academic studies?

Participants in this study included 1,014 nursing students and 58
graduate nurses with less than one year of practice. Six nursing schools,
representing three different programs of education—baccalaureate,
associate degree, and diploma—were involved. The investigation consisted of in-depth interviews of selected students from every year and
administration of the *Standard Measure of Inferences of Suffering*
questionnaire to all students in each school. Thus, the design of the
study included both longitudinal and cross-sectional aspects.

The *Standard Measure of Inferences of Suffering* questionnaire
used in all the studies consists of sixty items, describing a variety of patients with different illnesses and injuries. There are no right or wrong
answers. Subjects are asked to read each item and, on the basis of their
best judgment, to rate the patient on the degree of psychological
distress and physical pain they feel the patient experiences.

The extensive series of group interviews with approximately four to six students were held with all classes in each school. Because the data obtained from the interviews were primarily for exploratory purposes, the interviews were relatively unstructured and open-ended. Generally, the students were asked to discuss various aspects of their nursing education that influenced their reactions to patient suffering. They were also asked to describe how they believed their reactions had changed over the course of their education.

Findings

Analysis of the results of the responses to the *Standard Measure of Inferences of Suffering* questionnaire show that ratings of first-year, fall-term students differed significantly from all other groups. Ratings of physical pain and psychological distress decreased sharply between the fall and spring of the first year.

For both dimensions of suffering—physical pain and psychological distress—the most dramatic changes occurred during the first year. The changes for pain and psychological distress were in opposite directions. Inferences of physical pain decreased sharply between the fall and spring of the first year and then remained at about the same level throughout the entire program of education and during the first year of practice. In contrast, inferences of psychological distress increased sharply between the fall and spring of the first year and continued to rise during the second year. Thus, with regards to the central issue of this research, the data incontrovertibly show that inferences of suffering about patients are affected by education. Changes for the two aspects of suffering, physical pain and psychological distress, are in opposite directions. Inferences of patients' physical pain decrease in the course of nursing education; inferences of psychological distress, on the other hand, increase.

Several factors might account for these changes. Among the most important is the process of becoming acculturated within the subculture of nursing. As a result of contact with graduate students, faculty, clinical supervisors, students are exposed to beliefs these nurses hold

in common. Thus, through direct instruction, as well as through identification with nursing models, students acquire ways of thinking about
patient suffering.

For example, a senior nursing student said, "I've learned a lot
about patient suffering because of my instructors. They're role models
as teachers and as human beings. The way they talk to patients has
shown me a concern for people can be a very fulfilling part of life."

Another factor, of course, is simply that changes in students' inferences occur as a result of repeated exposure to patients who are suffering and the expectations that a student will respond as a professional. In our interviews with students, it was very clear that after the
first several months of fear and tension about suffering, students found
themselves becoming more objective and professional. They talked
about gaining control over their feelings. Others said they were surprised to find how quickly they learned not to feel scared or fearful. As
one nurse said, "You learn to tolerate patients' pain. You accept it as
something that has to be. I don't get upset. I can observe pain more ob-
jectively. I used to worry about asking patients if they had pain; now I
ask them questions and it doesn't bother me. As for myself, I'm more
tolerant about my own pain."

Others talked about how they had learned to set priorities, how
they have become more realistic, realizing there's only so much that can
be done about a person's pain. Fear drained away. Feeling scared or
upset disappeared. Repeatedly, students talked about how they had
rapidly learned to acquire self-control.

"I was pretty scared initially," one student reported. "Now I accept pain. Before, I didn't have a reference point about patients' pain. I
felt they all had a great deal of pain."

Another student agreed with this view, and added, "I'm a lot
more tolerant, able to curb my own anxieties so they don't interfere
with my work."

Insofar as physical pain was concerned, the students learned they
could manage, within limits, to cope with a patient's pain and discomfort. Medication could be given, the position of a patient could be
changed, and so forth. The lower ratings of pain by the students may

very well show that, as students go on in school, they learn that some physical pain relief measures are possible.

In contrast to the decrease in ratings for physical pain, ratings for psychological distress significantly increased. When we examined the curricula of the various schools, this finding is highly congruent with the emphasis on psychological understanding that was part of all the curricula. In every school, the psychological aspects of illness and management of pain were stressed. Students also noted that in their clinical courses, the instructors made a big point of their understanding the psychodynamics of each patient and how they affected the patient's condition.

The following comments reflect the fact that very early in training nursing students are sensitized to the psychological dimension of suffering.

"A lot of pain is fear, I've learned, so it's very important to understand a patient. I know with children they may not be as much in pain as scared, and this makes the pain worse. You can do a lot by understanding the patient and that's where psychology is so important. For example, a patient going up for surgery might have pain but much of the pain might also be anxiety, and talking to the patient and preparing them for surgery can help reduce the pain."

"The most important courses for me have been my communication courses and my 'psych' courses, including psychopathology."

"The psychological aspects of illness and pain have been stressed over and over. Our program is geared to a holistic approach to nursing."

"My courses and my instructors have made me a lot more aware of psychological aspects of suffering. I can accept the pain, but I think I'm more aware of what people are feeling."

"The whole first semester is devoted to how much patients need your attention. We have filmstrips, conferences, communication skills. A lot of stress is placed on psychology and sociology. I think we just realize how important the psychological aspects of a patient are."

"No matter if there isn't much pain, there's always some psychological distress in patients. I think we have to listen, ask questions, assess each situation. It depends on the patient, too; older people are lonely and there's a lot more psychological distress involved."

"I can remember crying with a dying person. I cried because I felt helpless. Now I'm less emotional. I do what I can. Now I can say to her, 'It's sad,' and offer support."

"The program has conditioned me to think about patients' psychological distress. As I get more experience, I understand more about the psychological aspects of illness."

"I'm aware that people can tolerate pain differently. I realize now that you can't help some patients' pain. Sometimes the best thing to do is just stay with the patient. The pain is relieved psychologically."

"I'm much more aware of psychological aspects. Before I started nursing school, I was kind and compassionate, but now I have so much more understanding of what goes on with patients."

"I've gained understanding that pain is a warning. I think that physical pain is a lot psychological. I know that if you talk to a patient before you do a procedure, they have less pain. My course work and my experience has made me more aware."

It is evident that as a consequence of their education, students are attuned to the psychological aspects of illness and indeed, consistently infer greater psychological distress than physical pain in evaluating the patients on the *Standard Measure of Inferences of Suffering* instrument.

The students who participated in this study came from three different types of programs: associate degree, diploma, and baccalaureate. There has been considerable discussion regarding the different types of students trained in these programs. We analyzed the data according to schools and the results show a similar pattern of change from entrance to graduation, regardless of the program. That is, whether a student was in a diploma school, an associate program, or a baccalaureate school, ratings of pain decreased and ratings of psychological distress increased by the end of the first year.

Examination of the curricula of the six schools studied, the reports of the students interviewed, and the changes in ratings of psychological distress over the course of training clearly demonstrate the enormous impact of both academic and clinical experiences on nursing students' beliefs about suffering. As a consequence of their education, nursing students are sensitized to the psychological dimension of suffering and indeed, consistently infer greater psychological distress than physical pain in evaluating the experiences of patients with a variety of illnesses or injuries.

The results of this research suggest that, while nursing education is highly successful in sensitizing prospective nurses to the psychological distress of patients, it may at the same time *desensitize* students to patients' pain. In nursing education during the past decade or so, there has been a great deal of effort devoted to increasing nurses' awareness of psychological factors involved in nursing care. Our findings indicate that, to a large extent, these efforts have succeeded insofar as nursing students' sensitivity to psychological distress is concerned. However, two problems suggest themselves in this context.

Having sensitized students to patients' psychological distress, it is not at all clear that nursing education also prepares nurses to deal effectively with this distress within the limitations confronted by most nurses in actual hospital practice. Given the demands of typical hospital environments, the time-consuming and emotionally demanding psychotherapeutically based techniques of dealing with psychological distress are often not practical, and sometimes not even possible. During training, with limited responsibilities and duties, nursing students may well have the opportunity to engage in extended conversations with their patients, gain empathic understanding, and provide psychological support. But in actual nursing practice, these opportunities are likely to be severely limited. Our observations of nurse-patient interactions reported in a preceding chapter indicate that the great majority of these interactions are very brief. Obviously, this is not a function of the nurses' insensitivity to patients' psychological distress; our research clearly points in exactly the opposite direction. Nurses are, by and large, very sensitive to the psychological dimensions of suffering. But given the exigencies of practice in most hospital situations, there is little opportunity to use effective techniques that demand a considerable amount of uninterrupted time and a good deal of energy. As a result, nurses who have been sensitized to patients' psychological distress may very well feel frustrated, and patients experiencing psychological distress may not receive the care that reduces it.

Thus, nursing education has successfully solved part of this general problem: nursing students are being sensitized to the psychological dimension of patient suffering. The second part of this problem involves the development of nursing techniques and procedures that effectively relieve patient distress and are practically feasible within the actual conditions of typical hospital practice. This part of the problem remains unsolved and presents a major challenge for future nursing reseach.

A second issue concerns the significant reduction in the amount of pain inferred by students as a consequence of their educational experiences. In a sense, student nurses are "taught" that patients feel less pain than these students believed patients did upon entering training. Perhaps this is an inevitable part of the process of what students during our interviews characterized as becoming "objective" or "professional." Indeed, it seems reasonable to expect a certain degree of emotional distancing between nurse and patient in the course of a student's professional development. As the students in our sample indicated, this distancing is not only desirable, but also necessary in order to function effectively in providing nursing care. But there may also be some potential danger in this educational process. Too much desensitization to patient pain, too much emotional distance between nurse and patient, too much reliance on routine procedures for relieving pain may significantly decrease the quality of nursing care. The present study does not provide a specific guideline to evaluate nursing education in these terms; however, the results suggest that nursing educators may profitably devote some attention to what their students are learning about patients' experiences of pain as well as psychological distress.

11

Nurses' Self-Reports about Their Reactions to Patient Suffering

A great deal of attention is always focused on patients' reactions to pain and illness. How do patients feel about hospitalization? What are patient experiences and reactions to their illnesses or injuries? We do not minimize the importance of these investigations; however, what about the experiences of nurses? What happens to nurses' judgments, emotional reactions, and personal attitudes in a profession that demands daily encounters with pain and distress?

We recall one incident in an emergency room. A severely injured child was brought in by ambulance. One of the attending nurses, a new graduate, burst into tears at the sight of the child. An ambulance attendant turned to her, "What gives?" he said with astonishment. "The kid's braver than you are. She's the one supposed to be crying—not the nurse."

Society sometimes expects nurses to be without feelings, without reactions. They're assumed to be 'above' all sorts of human feelings, for example, anger, dislike, apathy, irritation, depression, sadness, at least while they are on duty. It is occasionally forgotten that nurses are human, and, as they face problems dealing with the professional and human sides of nursing, they can, at times, be all "too human" in their responses.

In our investigations concerned with nurses' feelings, we asked several hundred nurses of varying ages, experience, religious and ethnic backgrounds, about their reactions to pain and distress of others, and what has happened to their attitudes from the time they first entered school to the time they had actually begun professional practice. In what ways did they think they had changed or remained the same in their response to patient suffering?

From School to Practice

Many of the nurses spoke about a shift from the idealism of school to the realism of practice, a shift from a kind of universal sympathy to more controlled and selective reactions.

"I know I don't feel the same toward patients now. . . . As a student, I think I cared more, because it was my whole life. Now I think I care differently because nursing is only part of my life. . . . In a way, I'm a better nurse. As a student, sometimes I felt my emotions kept me from behaving therapeutically."

"In school, I felt bad for everybody. A chest pain or a sore throat were all disasters. If someone said their throat was sore, I rushed around. Lie down, rest, gargle, I couldn't do enough for a complainer with a sore throat. Over time, I realized you have to react individually according to your own judgment."

"I know a lot of teachers in nursing schools teach that it's OK to cry with a patient if that's the way you feel. There's nothing wrong with showing emotion. But I feel since I've been in practice, restraint is important. You won't do the patient or the family any good if you stand there dissolved in your own tears."

Although most nurses talked about becoming more practical, realistic, and down-to-earth as a result of their professional experience, others reported an increased sensitivity to, and emotional understanding of, the suffering of others.

"Nursing education, at least for me, was a matter of studying, memorizing, and analyzing. I was so busy being a student, I didn't have time to feel. You have time to feel when you're in practice. I think, over time, I'm a far more sensitive and compassionate person than I was when I was in training."

"Practice has made me softer. I think I was more calloused as a student, probably because there was so much going on and you think in terms of labs and courses, not people."

Perhaps the two aspects of change that come about with practice—becoming more realistic and becoming more compassionate and understanding—are explained by the increased selectivity of nurses' reactions in contrast to the universal empathy of their nursing school experience.

"I can hear my instructor now, lecturing on how you can't get annoyed, you shouldn't ignore a patient. You have to feel empathy for everyone. Reality has taught me that I can't react to everyone in the same way."

"In nursing school, I was taught all patients have a certain equality. Regardless of the patient, I should have the same reactions. But patients are people—like the rest of the world. There are some I like and some I don't."

"When I first saw myself behaving differently, I got all upset. It wasn't right. But then, you can't just treat people the same. For example, my first emergency room experience. When I first worked in the unit, a patient would say 'I've been here for three hours.' I would rush around and demand the patient be seen. My goodness, no one should wait three hours! Now I see priorities. You can't start worrying about a sore throat in an emergency room when police are bringing in victims from an auto accident. The others can wait three hours, or four, if necessary. Some people are suffering more than others."

Differences in Reactions to Patients

Each nurse is especially sympathetic to certain kinds of patients. Some respond particularly to the young, some to the old, some to those who remind them of parents or friends.

"I think we all have favorite patients—people who trigger off a special feeling. I know that old people who don't complain get to me, and young kids, if they're not too way out in their behavior, and lonely patients. They make me feel something inside."

"Different kinds of people do turn you on. I mean, the fact is some people just get a rise out of you and others are just there to be taken care of. I get a different feeling when someone my own age comes in, or someone who reminds me of my parents, or even friends."

The nature of the illness makes a tremendous difference in the nurses' reactions. They respond most strongly to those who are likely to die or be severely disabled. By and large, less sympathy is felt for patients with minor illnesses, and those who don't have a 'legitimate' complaint.

"Most nurses I know are more torn apart when they work with young patients who have serious illnesses. Young people are very disturbing. It isn't fair they should suffer. I feel for the parents. I guess I could compare my feelings for parents of children in for tonsillectomies. If they carry on, I turn off. But when I have a seriously ill child with concerned parents, the situation can be traumatizing."

"I just can't feel the same for a patient who, let's say, has appendicitis and one who has cancer. They are different and I know the person who is 'postop' for appendicitis might have pain; still in all, I really feel bad for the person who has cancer."

"I just couldn't feel anything for this woman, even though she had a great deal of pain. This was her sixth operation for beauty's sake. When she complained, I couldn't see her pain being real. She did it to herself for her appearance. I know I made her wail before I responded."

Sometimes the nurse's own personal experiences make a significant difference in her response to particular patients. Having gone through similar experiences, a nurse may be especially sensitive or "tuned in" to a patient's suffering.

"Before I had a baby, I worked in labor and delivery. We'd have these women carrying on as if the world were coming to an end. 'Come on now,' I felt like telling them. 'You're putting on a show.' Well, let me tell you, I had a baby and I had a difficult labor. You ought to see me now on the floor. All that a woman has to do is squeak about her pain and I empathize right with her."

"Not long ago, I had an abdominal operation—nothing serious, but I doubled over in pain for a day or so. Recently I had a young patient who had the same kind of 'postop' pain. I was very sympathetic. . . . Every time he complained, I was right there. I doubt if I would have shown the same kind of consideration if I hadn't had a similar experience."

For most nurses, a feeling of sympathy for the patient leads to increased contact with that patient. They are more likely to stop in and just chat. In contrast, there is much less conversation with patients for whom they feel little sympathy. By and large, the amount of conversation a nurse has with a patient is probably a good indicator of the degree of sympathy the nurse feels for that person.

"With patients I feel something for, I'll talk about anything. I can always find something to talk about. With someone I don't feel anything for, I don't even talk about the weather. I simply say, 'Do this or that'—I keep the conversation to a minimum."

"When I go in to a patient for whom I just can't feel much of a reaction, I don't say more than I have to. I feel guilty, because the patient will sometimes try to talk and my responses are terse. I say just what is necessary—not a word more."

Nurses realize that it is not merely what you say to a patient that makes a difference, but how you say it.

"When you care about a patient . . . it comes through in your tone."

"I know from myself and listening to other nurses that something changes when you talk to patients you care about and to those you don't. When you sympathize with a patient, I think—I know I do—you speak more slowly. There's a tenderness in your voice. You don't run out of the room. If the patient wants to talk, you stay and talk. Or maybe you don't talk at all because you don't know what to say, but there's something in your face that lets the patient know you're pulling for him."

"Something happens to you when you're with patients you feel a lot for. I think it's like a wave of gentleness or tenderness. It sweeps over you when you care. I suppose I show in my voice and hands. I know that inside I feel warm and soft. I'm sure I do something to express that feeling."

Nurses have certain expectations regarding patients who have a "right" to complain, and those who are merely "complainers." There is a crucial difference between those patients whom the nurse believes are really suffering and those who are seen as overacting and complaining simply for the sake of complaining. Continuous complaints, if they are seen as unwarranted, are frustrating. For the nurse constantly faced with these complaints, irritation, annoyance, and anger are not uncommon responses.

"I feel I know who is sick and who is making a noise. Then I realize I treat people who I feel are really sick different from the way I do people who are just making a noise."

"When I don't feel sympathy for a patient simply because I know they are not really suffering, I still do what I have to in terms of care, but I think I sound angry. I know I stay at the foot of the bed of those people. I never go up to the head of the bed. I hear myself talking a mile a minute and then I walk out without waiting for an answer."

"When I don't feel a patient is really in pain or has some kind of emotional problem and keeps calling for a nurse, I get annoyed. I mean, there are patients who really need me. Then you have one who doesn't need you but constantly puts on his light. When this happens I know I take my time to answer. Of course I eventually go in, but I go what I call a roundabout way. I don't hurry. I just go on down the hall like I'm out for an afternoon stroll. I do what I have to and then I leave the room quickly. I don't linger with those kinds of patients. . . ."

In addition to feeling angry, the nurses typically avoid the complainer. Some nurses delay their responses; others respond, but don't hear what the patient says.

"If I think a patient is putting on a light just for the usual complaint, I don't think I see it. I'm not conscious of the light."

"There are some patients I don't hear. I know they're talking and asking questions, but I can't hear a word they say."

Nurses may or may not express their anger openly, but when they recognize their own feelings, they frequently report a sense of guilt.

"I feel guilty because I know the patient is sick and maybe not responsible for his actions. I can't help not liking the patient, but I also feel guilty. Then I go into the patient's room and try to make it up to him."

"I resent the patient and then I rush around bringing him this and that, and I get angry at myself and angry at the patient."

"I may lecture to patients. I know when I go into a long harangue about what the patient should do, I'm trying to make up for negative feelings."

Dealing with Emotional Problems

For some nurses not involved in psychiatric nursing, patients with emotional problems tend to elicit relatively little sympathy.

"I guess I don't feel much sympathy for people with psychiatric problems. I mean, they come in neurotic, all upset, and self-centered. I don't want to take care of them."

"Of course I take care of these people. I give them attention and I try to sympathize with their problems, but deep down inside of me, I wonder about why they can't get on top of their problems."

Part of the nurses' difficulty in dealing with emotional problems is their feelings of helplessness or inadequacy in relieving this kind of suffering. They can administer medication to reduce physical pain, but they don't have similarly effective and efficient techniques for relieving psychological distress.

"I know what to do with the patient physically. I can give pain medications and treatment, but when it comes to saying the right comforting words, I feel at a loss. I can understand a patient's tension, but I find it hard to tolerate."

"It's so much easier to cope with physical pain than psychological suffering. If someone has physical pain, you can do something and you see the results. I know that's why I prefer the recovery room to the 'med-surg' floor. I feel satisfied when I can help. But on other units, you have to handle physical pain and psychological problems. I have compassion. I feel for most of the patients, but honestly, I haven't any idea what is best to do. If someone is depressed or disturbed, what do you say? What can you do? You can't handle it the way you handle physical pain."

"We studied psychological theories and counseling techniques, but in practice you don't sit down with a patient for an hour a week or an hour every day. . . . Nowhere in school did they tell me how to be therapeutic in five minutes. We do have to work on schedules."

"As a student, I never thought about psychological needs except in psychology classes. But now I'm more aware and concerned. It bothers me that I can't do more to help patients who have psychological problems."

The Problem of Over-involvement

Far more common than the problem of avoiding complainers is the other side of the coin—the nurse's sense of being overwhelmed by the very real suffering of patients she works with every day. Nurses described a variety of reactions to this stress, including, for example, the empathic development of physical symptoms that parallel those of a particular patient.

"I had this one patient I was caring for on the floor for several months. I really felt for this patient, and there were times when I actually felt like I had the same symptoms. I really had chest pains. They were so bad I had myself checked out. Nothing was wrong, and I realize now that I was so upset about the patient that I started to get the same kind of pains she had."

"Lots of times, when I have patients that really upset me because they're in such pain or maybe depressed or worried, I get physical reactions. I've had headaches. Then there was this woman with thrombophlebitis in her legs, and she was suffering terribly. I remember feeling my legs hurt whenever I had to go into her room."

The effects of daily experience with the suffering of others is not only felt at work. Nurses often reported that they took patients' problems home with them.

"I'm drained when I get home. If I've spent a day feeling for other people, I get frustrated. My family gets the worst side of me. I can get explosive, angry, and when someone at home sounds off about being sick or worried, I get resentful. I ask myself, who is going to listen to my aches and pains?"

"If you feel too much at work you just don't want to feel when you go home. You've had it."

"I have to work at seeing good in life. I see so much that is sad and negative that I have to work at feeling positive. I think seeing so much suffering affects my life. I do know I need to get lots of different stimuli when I get away from the hospital."

"I have lost contact with old friends. Now I'm more comfortable with the people in medicine. They have more to say to me. You see, I feel as a nurse I've touched the real core of life. This makes you wake up. Other people can go along and never see what I see. I grew up in practice, far more than friends my own age who aren't nurses."

"If you like being a nurse, it's twenty-four hours a day, whether you like it or not. I have called co-workers at night to talk about a patient who worried me."

For many nurses, some time after they begin practicing, they realize the need to develop some emotional distance between themselves and their work, some defense for them against over-involvement.

"I think you have to block out some of the patients' suffering. If I reacted to every patient, felt deeply, I couldn't exist outside of the hospital—or in the hospital, for that matter."

"You can't go around weeping and crying with patients. A job has to be done."

"I couldn't take the pain and suffering when I first started to work. My work history is horrible; one year on and one year off, or sometimes three months at a stretch. It's better now, but simply because I've built up some defenses."

Frequently, the need for emotional distance developed as a result of experience with a patient for whom the nurse felt especially sympathetic and who subsequently died, leaving the nurse feeling drained, traumatized, and ineffective.

"I was very tired. Taking care of him had been very exhausting, emotionally and physically. I realized later I shouldn't get attached this way, for my own sake. The next couple of weeks I kept a certain distance between myself and other patients. If I didn't, I know I couldn't give the kind of physical care they needed. Giving so much of yourself emotionally interferes with physical care."

"You have to be careful about focusing on one patient. You can't get too close. It happened to me once and I realized how bad it was. The patient was a little girl, and when she died I was so broken up that I couldn't work."

Thus, to maintain their own emotional stability and remain effective in professional practice, nurses build psychological defenses against over-involvement. These defenses typically involve establishing some emotional distance. But specific defensive reactions take many forms, including, for example, seemingly macabre but psychologically meaningful hospital humor.

"There's only so much you can feel, so much you can see. You have to escape, and I guess you can say that cracking jokes is an escape."

"I think we (nurses) build up defenses about suffering. I think we depend on humor. Maybe it isn't humor—more like black comedy. I know there are some awful situations when people make jokes. To an outsider, the humor seems terrible, but in the hospital it's funny. I guess humor seems terrible, but in the hospital it's funny. I guess humor helps you cope."

Reactions to Death and Dying

Of all the daily problems encountered by nurses, the death of a patient is emotionally the most devastating. Even after years of professional experience, nurses described their reactions to the death of a patient with whom they had worked in terms of feelings of helplessness, depression, anger, and despair.

"I was caught up with the patient. He was in terrible pain and very worried about his family. He didn't ask for anything—just lay there staring. I tried to get him to talk, but he shook his head; and yet I had the idea he wanted me to stay in the room. I felt awful. Inside, the pit of my stomach felt ripped. I was nauseated."

"Another nurse and I were taking care of a young man we knew was going to die in a few days. The whole staff was shook up. When he died, we broke down completely. I remember we just went to the lounge and sat there crying. All that day if someone looked at us, or if we looked at each other, tears came to our eyes. It was awful. We couldn't stop crying."

"When I was a student it was a lark—I was going to help people. I was young and had never seen a person die or a baby being born. It was a game I was playing. Now it's real. In school, we were protected from even death. I can recall how we (students) were rushed away one afternoon because a patient was dying. Now each day I see more, and it's depressing."

"I keep asking myself, what did I do? What didn't I see? Couldn't anything have been done?"

The death of young people is especially traumatic for many nurses.

"I was taking care of a young woman who should never have died. She was demanding and kept calling me on the intercom. One afternoon, she asked me to call her husband; she just wanted to know if he was okay. I got upset myself because, when she was dying, I started to cry—couldn't control myself. The supervisor got enraged. She said to me, 'You have no business crying. This isn't the first and last patient you will take care of.' I keep thinking, even now, what right did she have to say that to me? Tell me how to feel? When she died, I couldn't touch the body. I could look but not touch her. I was too shaken. The day nurses came in and washed the body I stayed away from the room."

"It makes me angry when a child dies. Why should a child die? Why should a young person die? I can't answer, and it bothers me a lot."

When a patient with whom the nurse has been closely involved is dying, a common reaction reported is a desire to escape from the situation, though physical escape itself often does not relieve the nurse's own sense of emotional distress.

"She wanted desperately to live. She was in a tent, and when you went near the bed, she would grab you by the wrist. She hadn't energy to eat by herself, but her grip was unbelievable. She kept saying, 'I don't want to die. I don't want to die.' I couldn't bear going into the room."

"I just couldn't go in anymore after I knew she was going to die. I did anything I could just to get out of going in her room."

The trauma of death is reduced somewhat when the patient is elderly and the nurse senses that the person is "ready to die."

"A 77-year-old man was very sweet to the end. He told us how he felt. 'I'm ready to die,' he said. 'I wish they'd let me go in peace.' He was easy to care for. I wasn't helpless. We prayed together. But, as he said, 'My job in the world is done.' I just loved talking to him. All the nurses did. He was very calm. He asked us to shave him and help him get dressed. Imagine, and he died that afternoon. It was as if he knew that the hour was coming and he wanted to be clean and ready. I knew I had helped him—had stayed with him, done things—and I was glad that I had been able to be supportive."

"There is less of a reaction when an old person dies. It's not that I don't feel as much, but I feel differently. There was a 76-year-old man recently, and he had a loving family—six children—and he had lived a full life. He told me he was ready to die. He said that he had lived a good life and his children were all fine, and his grandchildren, too. He was tired of suffering. I didn't feel as bad about him."

In addition to the nurses' immediate emotional reactions, the experience of death of a patient also affects the nurses' thoughts and feelings about her own death and her reflections about herself and her life.

"I feel empty inside; part of me is gone and not coming back. Each time this happens, I get a new awareness of myself as an individual who is also going to die. Then I say to myself, what I do in life from day to day is very important. If anything, encounters with death have increased my self-awareness."

"Over time, awareness of my own mortality has hit me. I'm a little nicer to myself. I take myself out to dinner and get a treat. I used to be worried about the future and if something didn't work out, I was impossible. Now I don't worry as much. It's all right if something doesn't work out."

"The spectre of death is in the hospital. The time factor of life bothers me. As a student, you plan for the future. You think in terms of saving, then in practice, you wake up to the fact that you can't save some people. When I hear the call of one-two-six, I shudder—I feel terrible. I realize I don't want to die."

The comments of the nurses and the implications of what they said raise many questions about nursing education and practice. We cannot hope to touch all of the issues raised and we certainly don't intend even to suggest possible solutions. But we would like to underscore some of the central issues discussed, and perhaps suggest some questions that might be considered in dealing with these issues.

Many young people enter nursing with a strong sense of idealism that is reflected in a kind of universal sympathetic reaction to everyone who is suffering. This is certainly a very positive motivation for nurses, and, in certain respects, it would be highly desirable to maintain this sense of idealism throughout a nurse's professional career.

But, for some nurses at least, the realities of practice provide a sharp jolt to this idealism. They cannot spend time with everyone who complains; they cannot relieve the suffering of every patient; they do not feel honestly sympathetic towards everyone; they cannot prevent death in every case. Thus, the initial idealism of their nursing school days is inevitably modified.

In itself, this process of modification is not necessarily undesirable. Nevertheless, one cannot help but wonder about the degree to which nursing school experiences might foster an idealism that is incongruent with practice. With the recent emphasis on psychological understanding of the patient, has there also been an adequate parallel emphasis on understanding the nurse? Do students learn that nurses, too, are people, and that no person can like or feel sympathetic toward everyone? Is it always wrong for a nurse to feel angry? Should nurses feel guilty when they can't respond sympathetically? How do nurses' feelings influence the effectiveness of nursing care? What can nursing schools do differently to bridge the gap between idealism and the reality of practice, between the professional and human sides of being a nurse?

Nurses see a clear distinction between relieving physical pain and comforting a patient in psychological distress. For relief of pain, medications and other physical techniques are available and relatively effective—certainly more consistently effective than the psychological techniques currently used to deal with emotional distress. Thus, nurses have more difficulty responding to psychological aspects of suffering than to physical pain.

This difficulty arises primarily because effective and efficient techniques for reducing psychological distress are not readily available. As the nurses in this study pointed out, a staff nurse working in a typical large hospital isn't able to spend long daily sessions with each patient, searching for profound, in-depth insights and psychological understanding.

The differences between psychotherapeutic and general nursing situations are enormous, and perhaps the theories and techniques developed for psychotherapy are inappropriate sources for the task facing a nurse. In most nonpsychiatric situations, the nurse needs to relieve immediate emotional distress. What sources are more appropriate for the development of such techniques? Instead of searching for other sources, would it be more profitable for nurses and nursing researchers to focus on the problems and situations specific to nursing and develop techniques particularly suitable to the typical nurse-patient interaction?

The nurses in this study dramatically described the dangers of over-involvement with particular patients. In fact, it was often an experience of over-involvement with a specific patient that led the nurse to realize that deeply personal and emotional reactions can interfere with one's effective functioning on the job.

Many nurses reported dealing with this problem by developing a degree of emotional distance from the patients. But this, too, involves dangers and difficulties. From the patients' point of view, the nurses may be seen as uncaring, rejecting, and mechanical, adding to a patients' sense of loneliness and helplessness. From the nurses' point of view, work may lose some of the human quality that originally attracted them to nursing. As a result, nurses may become increasingly dissatisfied and even bored by the more routine and administrative tasks that permit them to maintain a certain emotional distance from the patient.

Nurses have been concerned with this problem for a very long time, and there is no easy solution. Nevertheless, there are questions that need to be explored, and perhaps in the process of exploration, a more adequate solution to this central conflict in nursing will be developed. For example, what is the relationship between emotional distance and nursing effectiveness? Is a sense of sympathetic involvement with the patients a condition of effective nursing care? In what ways does the structure of the hospital situation itself exacerbate this problem? How do the nurses' working relationships with other professionals influence their relationships with patients? In what ways can the situation be altered to improve the interpersonal conditions of nursing for both the nurse and the patient?

Of all the problems discussed by the nurses participating in this study, their reactions to death and dying of patients clearly elicited the strongest emotional responses. We cannot meaningfully add to what nurses have already said with such clear emotional force. Perhaps the only conclusion that needs to be drawn is a reaffirmation of the necessity to continue, and even expand, our concern for those who face the fact of mortality in their everyday professional lives.

12

From An Administrator's Perspective

Charlene Fischi Rubin, B.S.N.E., M.A., Me.D.

Dealing with patients' suffering, both in terms of pain and psychological distress, is obviously a central issue in nursing, and therefore, a primary concern of nursing administrators. The nursing administrator is in a unique position to receive information about nurse-patient relationships from several points of view: reports from patients, nurses, doctors, and other hospital personnel.

Having been in nursing administration for many years, I have handled numerous problems concerned with nurse-patient relationships. After reviewing the research contained in this book, I can see that, in retrospect, the responses to patients expressed by my nursing staff can, in part, be explained by the belief systems nurses have about patient pain and distress.

In general, it has been my experience that seriously ill patients and their families have felt the nursing care exemplary. However, patients admitted for diagnostic or elective purposes, patients who constantly express a great deal of pain, demand considerable attention, and who are emotional about their conditions receive much less positive reactions from the nursing staff.

Repeatedly, nurses have told me that they do not like caring for patients who treat nurses in a condescending manner; for example, saying to the nurse, "Would you be a sweetheart and get me some fresh water?" Nurses prefer caring for patients who need professional care or who really appreciate everything a nurse does for them. Several nurses have commented, "After all, we're professional nurses, not maids." Others react negatively to patients who fit the demanding, complaining stereotype. These patients only want doctors' advice and instructions and feel the nurse can't teach them anything.

The research reported in this volume suggests that nurses tend to discount the suffering of these overly demanding, complaining patients. Thus, the nurse may pay even less attention to the patients' complaints, and this of course leads to increasing patient dissatisfaction.

As every administrator knows, not a day passes without patient complaints about indifferent nursing behaviors. The special responsibility of the administrator is to serve as an objective mediator in these situations. The following examples illustrate typical situations I have encountered in my role as a nursing administrator.

Case 1

The nursing supervisor, Ms. Morgan, received a complaint from Ms. Smith that she was not receiving her pain medication and was not being properly treated for her diarrhea. At the same time, Ms. Smith's husband called me and further recounted his wife's dissatisfaction with the nursing care. He told me he was certain the nurses did not like his wife. "They make her wait and wait before answering the light. They stand at the nurses' station and laugh about her diarrhea."

I called the supervisor and asked her to please investigate this complaint and report the results to me. The comprehensive report showed that the nurses felt that Ms. Smith was a very demanding patient, as well as a management problem. The nurses' notes seemed to bear this out. For example, one note stated, "Those kinds of people are never satisfied."

From the point of view of the nurses, Ms. Smith wasn't really suffering, but was merely demanding. From Ms. Smith's perspective, she was experiencing considerable discomfort and feeling rejected by the staff. In this case, we were able to resolve the problem by involving everyone concerned—the nurses, the patient, and the supervisor. Through lengthy discussions, the nursing staff gained some insight into their personal feelings, and Ms. Smith recognized that her pain medication was no longer a primary concern. The heart of the problem was her belief that the nurses didn't accept her pain. Once she realized that the nurses were not making a joke about her, Ms. Smith recognized that her pain medication was no longer the central issue. What was really important to her was that the nurses were trying to alleviate her pain and that they paid more attention to her personally.

Case 2

Contrary to the old nursing philosophy, the new look in nursing is that all nurses cannot care for all patients. The nurse, as well as the patient, is a unique individual, and as the following case demonstrates, situations may arise where the nurses' judgments about a suffering patient may interfere with the nurse-patient relationship.

Ms. Sunderland, a patient, called my office to complain about a nurse's "poor attitude" and "brusque manner." The night supervisor investigated the complaint and reported that the patient, in a haughty and unpleasant manner, had asked the nurse to remove the bedpan. The nurse stated, "Ms. Sunderland always addressed me in this tone, as if I were a servant or something. When I entered the room for routine rounds, she angrily asked me what I was looking for. I personally haven't done anything to provoke her anger. I think she is a resentful person who doesn't want to remain on bedrest."

The nurse, according to the night supervisor, had a casual manner toward this patient's expressions of discomfort. Similar situations had occurred, and efforts to get the nurse to show more concern were never successful. The nurse remained casual and brusque. The supervisor reported that the nurse had said she could not and would not change her personality for anyone.

Since the patient did not want to see the nurse in her room again, it was considered advisable to reassign the nurse to another patient. In certain instances, the nursing administrator can help an individual nurse function more effectively regarding a patient's suffering by recognizing that the interests of the patient as well as the nurse sometimes necessitate shifting the patient to another unit or reassigning the nurse to another patient.

Case 3

The patient, Mrs. Williams, complained that she had to wait forever for the nurse to answer her light. "What if I really were here for an emergency? For this kind of money, I should get more service."

The supervisor checked the complaint and reported to me that the incident occurred only once, during an evening when the unit was at its peak of activity. The nursing staff were irate with Mrs. Williams. Several stated that, "She's a real nut. She doesn't want to care for herself. Even the doctors think she's a pain in the neck. All she really wants is to find out what happened to the patients down the hall. She's constantly seeking attention from the staff. She never has visitors. Her husband has only come once. She hasn't complained before because, whenever possible, we would sit and listen to her many problems."

This case illustrates a common problem nurses face. From their point of view, the patient is overly reacting to hospitalization. From the patient's point of view, she is suffering from considerable psychological distress. The task facing the administrative staff is to help the nurses see how their judgments might influence their nursing care. In this instance, counseling sessions for the staff helped them to understand Mrs. Williams's strong needs for attention, stemming from her extreme psychological distress.

Case 4

Mr. Gianetti, a patient, called the hospital administrator to complain about his nursing care. He very loudly and angrily stated that if something wasn't done, he would sign himself out of the hospital. His complaints were that the nurses were "very bossy," and ordered him about as if he were a child.

When questioned, the staff stated that Mr. Gianetti refused to remain on bedrest, smoked in his bed, using the urinal and bed sheets as ashtrays, wouldn't take any of his medications, and was very noisy.

The charge nurse and supervisor sat down with Mr. Gianetti to discuss his complaints and to determine how the staff might best meet his nuring care needs. During the discussion, Mr. Gianetti softened his manner and agreed to become more amenable to the plan of care *if* the nurses would "stop ordering me around and let me make some of my own decisions. After all, it's my health, not theirs. I'm the kind of man who never gets sick and is not used to women pushing me around. I make my own decisions. Is that clear? Now what do you want me to do?"

In this case, the patient's resentment of his dependency in the hospital provoked the nurses to behave in a somewhat more authoritarian manner than they might otherwise have done, and this authoritarian behavior led to even greater resentment on the part of the patient. An important part of the nursing administrator's responsibility is to help the nursing staff gain greater awareness and understanding of these kinds of difficulties, and on the basis of this understanding, break the vicious cycle of resentment and counter-resentment in nurse-patient interactions.

Case 5

Several studies in this research considered judgments of patient distress as a function of the patients' cultural backgrounds. The findings showed that nurses' judgments about patient suffering were influenced by the patients' cultural backgrounds. The following written complaint came into my office; it considers this very issue from the patient's perspective.

> I am a medical recording clerk. Recently I was a surgical patient in my own hospital. About the personnel and the care I received in Westwood Pavillion, I have only positive feelings. I am writing to you because of my brief but traumatic experience in the recovery room. My

operative procedure was relatively minor, but the results were quite painful. The surgeon excised scar tissue from a poorly healed rectal fissure as well as the resultant thrombosed rectal tag. I awoke abruptly in the recovery room because I had a feeling of urgency. Initially I was disoriented. I thought I was still in the holding room. I expressed my urgency aloud and I was promptly assisted onto a bedpan. At that point, I felt a sharp pain. I then asked to be taken to the bathroom because I thought my inability to go on to the bedpan had changed my urgency to pain. I was told that I was in the recovery room and that I could only use the bedpan and not the bathroom.

Suddenly I felt wide awake, and I looked at the clock on the wall. It was 2 P.M. I realized that I had already been operated on and that the pain was becoming more intense. The nurse told me I had to wait until I was brought back to the floor.

For the next half hour, I went up and back between moaning for someone to take me back to the floor and shifting my body from side to side to get into a less uncomfortable position. I wanted to scream, but I did not want to disturb the other patients. During that time, a nurse asked me to stop shifting because I was dislodging my dressing. I was also asked by the clerk at the desk if I wasn't a hospital employee. I said, "Yes," and she asked me why I was acting that way. The nurse smiled and added to this remark that I wasn't behaving like "a typical Oriental patient." I did not answer them. I was trying to cope with the most intense pain I have ever felt.

Since I received a "Stat" dose of Demerol when I returned to the floor, I assume there was no medical reason for denial of medication in the recovery room. At a time when I needed support and comfort, I was subjected to non-supportive comments about not living up to model Oriental behavior, which only increased my discomfort.

I feel a need to get this off my chest, but I also feel that no one else, employees or not, should feel traumatized by a stay in any unit of our Hospital. Thank you for your time and listening to my complaints.

Sincerely yours,
Ake Yung

In this case, the nurses' reactions to the patient's distress appeared to be influenced by the patient's ethnic background. Recognizing that these kinds of biases may affect our judgments is a first step in correcting the bias, thus allowing the nurse to respond to the individual **patient rather than a general stereotype.**

Case 6

The patient, Sheila Green, complained that when the night nurse answered the buzzer, her sharp response was limited to asking, "What do you want?" Ms. Green said that this happened on several occasions when she needed pain medication. She described the nurse as "Indian, very unpleasant, insensitive, and never smiling."

According to the supervisor, the nurse, Ms. Ram, was an Asian woman who spoke with a British accent. She suggested that Ms. Ram's unfamiliar accent and inflection could be misinterpreted as sharp by Ms. Green. Although she felt that Ms. Ram's personal manner might appear abrupt, she considered Ms. Ram to be a very conscientious nurse.

On the other hand, the supervisor added, Ms. Green was known to everyone as a complainer, especially in reference to pain medication. "As a matter of fact," the supervisor noted, "Ms. Green has told me that her doctors have not been telling her what is really wrong with her. They do not order enough medication to relieve her pain. On one occasion, I walked into her room and overheard her phone conversation with her lawyer. Her complaints have all been documented."

This case again reflects a problem resulting from cultural differences. From the nurse's point of view, Ms. Green was not in constant pain, and therefore, had no real need for pain medication. From Ms. Green's perspective, she was in considerable pain. In this case, it proved extremely helpful to have a conference with the nurse and the patient in order to bridge the cultural differences. When Ms. Ram understood that Ms. Green's expressions of pain were very real for her, she could care for the patient without feeling that Ms. Green was an unreasonably demanding woman.

Case 7

Mr. Andrew Jackson came to the nursing office to lodge a complaint about the nursing care on his unit. He reported that "even the head nurse did not listen to my complaints." He stated that when he requested clean pajamas and linen, the nurse told him, "You should go to the Waldorf Astoria."

The supervisor submitted the following report:

> Mr. Jackson has been a patient at this hospital many times. He has psoriasis and G.U. problems. It seems that Mr. Jackson wants a clean pair of pajamas after each shower. When we ran out of pajamas, we offered him a patient gown. This made him very angry, and he yelled that we were treating him as an inferior. He also wants his bed changed after each shower. He frequently was not in his bed and the staff did change the sheets. This is when the nurse said, "They don't even change the sheets in the Waldorf Astoria three times a day." Although I have tried to explain to Mr. Jackson why we can't always accommodate his laundry wishes, he still holds fast to his belief that "private" patients should be treated better than other patients in the hospital.
>
> I spoke with the nurse about her unnecessary response concerning the Waldorf. She admitted the remark was inappropriate but deserving.

In dealing with this problem from an administrative point of view, it was important to communicate to the patient the realistic limits of hospital care. On the other hand, it was equally important to help the nursing staff recognize and appreciate the basis of the patient's demands, and to work out a solution that took into account the patient's discomfort, but at the same time was realistic in terms of the resources available.

Recommendations

Whenever I have discussed patient complaints with nurses, they would frequently attribute the problems to poor staffing, insufficient supplies and equipment, and not having enough time to meet the "demands of recalcitrant patients." They also maintained that the hospital administration never supported them and always assumed that the nurses had antagonized the patients. Certainly some of these factors may contribute to unsatisfactory nurse-patient relationships. However, despite this fact, we cannot lose sight of the fact that "understanding the process of how we judge patient suffering is extremely important. Knowledge gives us the capacity to understand others and ourselves. We have found that as we increasingly understand the cultural distances between provider and consumer we can begin to alter case delivery in order to reduce this distance.''[1]

The task for the nursing administrator is to help nurses function more effectively regarding patient suffering. Some of the ways this can be accomplished are as follows:

1. Scheduling of unit conferences that include all members of the health care team to discuss pain and distress and the ways people react to suffering.

2. Routine counseling sessions for staff members who feel physically and emotionally drained.

3. Discussions with nurses to help them recognize their own feelings toward individual patients and encourage a more understanding and tolerant approach.

4. Reassigning nurses to other patients when differences cannot be resolved between the nurse and the patient. In some instances, I have found it necessary to transfer a patient to another unit.

5. Improvements of the work situation, which are bound to have a positive effect on nurses' behaviors. Although staffing, supplies, and equipment do not directly enter nurses' judgments about patient suffering, we must also recognize that the working situation can affect a nurse's tolerance toward a demanding patient.

6. Periodic review by the administrator of factors and findings that influence nurses' judgments about patient suffering, so that the staff can be alerted.

I have found that a strong program of continuing education and in-service classes can be extremely valuable for this purpose.

---

[1]Ingeborg G. Mauksch, Nursing Issues Surrounding Health Care Delivery, *Journal of Nursing Education* 9(June 1978): 1-15.

13
Some Thoughts for the Future

In the research we have discussed in this book, we have dealt with two aspects of nurses' beliefs about patients: the degree of psychological distress patients experience and the amount of pain they feel. We have found that nurses more or less share common beliefs about patient suffering and these beliefs are related to the ways in which nurses care for patients. This represents an important step in furthering our understanding of nursing practice, but there is obviously much more that can be done to gain a fuller understanding of those factors that contribute to meaningful nurse-patient relationships.

Further investigations might well consider other aspects of nurses' beliefs relevant to patient care. For example, it would be useful to know more about nurses' beliefs regarding the degree to which patients are responsible for their own illnesses or injuries. In our work with nurses who participated in this research we observed, from time to time, differences in nurses' behaviors that apparently stemmed from their beliefs about patients' responsibilities for their conditions. For example, in working with drug addicts or alcoholics, those nurses who believed that patients were largely responsible for their own conditions behaved differently toward these patients in contrast to nurses who did not share this belief. Behavioral differences reflecting nurses' attitudes seemed to be true not only for drug addiction and alcoholism, but also for other illnesses and injuries. Therefore, to expand our understanding of nursing practice, studying nurses' beliefs about patient responsibility would be extremely helpful.

Another related concern that might be investigated is nurses' beliefs about what patients are capable of doing. If a nurse believes a patient is unable to learn certain basic techniques of health care, the nurse's educational efforts may be sharply curtailed. Conversely, if a nurse believes a patient is able to learn, the nurse may very well intensify efforts to educate the patient. The following example illustrates the difference in behaviors of two nurses who differed in their beliefs about the ability of a diabetic patient to accept instruction regarding his diet. According to one nurse, the patient was "hopeless." She felt her repeated efforts to go over the diet were a waste of time because the patient simply refused to respond to her teaching. The other nurse, however, felt that, eventually, the patient's resistance to teaching would break down. As a consequence of her conviction that the message eventually would get through to the patient, she stepped up her teaching efforts.

A third related area involves nurses' beliefs about the effectiveness of various therapeutic measures. For example, one might explore nurses' beliefs about the effects of psychological support on a patient's condition. The nurse who believes that extensive psychological support can make a difference in the patient's well-being may expend more effort in relating to that patient, for example involving the family or providing extra attention. The nurse who tends to discount the psychological components of illness may not build these factors into the nursing care plan.

These examples represent only a few areas of belief that might be investigated. As we acquire more knowledge about the many aspects of nurses' belief systems and how these beliefs are related to nursing behaviors, we will understand more fully the fundamental basis of nursing. In caring for patients, a nurse confronts an enormous variety of complex and potentially significant stimuli that she must selectively perceive and interpret. In part, the selective perceptions and interpretations a nurse makes are influenced by her belief systems. Our research has demonstrated that nurses' belief systems are tied to behavior; therefore, it would seem extremely important to investigate the belief systems in a wide variety of areas in order to build a systematic foundation for effective nursing care.

Bibliography

Baer, E., Davitz, L. J., and R. Lieb. Inferences of physical pain and psychological distress in relation to verbal and nonverbal patient communication. *Nursing Research* 19 (September–October 1970), 388–392.

Beecher, H. K. *Measurement of Subjective Responses.* New York: Oxford University Press, 1959.

Burnside, H., Davitz, L. J., and C. B. Lenburg. Inferences of physical pain and psychological distress in relation to length of time in the nursing education program. *Nursing Research* 19 (September–October 1970), 399–401.

Copp, L. A. The spectrum of suffering. *American Journal of Nursing* 74: (1974) 491–495.

Davitz, L. J. and J. R. Davitz. How do nurses feel when patients suffer? *American Journal of Nursing* 75:9 (1975), 1505–1510.

Davitz, L. J. and J. R. Davitz. How nurses view patient suffering. *R.N.* (October 1975).

Davitz, L. J. and S. H. Pendelton. Nurses' inferences of suffering, Study 1: Cultural differences. *Nursing Research* 18 (March–April 1969), 100–103.

Davitz, L. J. and S. H. Pendelton. Nurses' inferences of suffering, Study 2: Clinical specialties. *Nursing Research* 18 (March–April 1969), 103–105.

Davitz, L. J. and S. H. Pendelton. Nurses' inferences of suffering, Study 3: Patient diagnosis. *Nursing Research* 18 (March–April 1969), 104–105.

Davitz, L. J. and S. H. Pendelton. Nurses' inferences of suffering, Study 4: Patient characteristics. *Nursing Research* 18 (March–April 1969), 105–107.

Davitz, L. J., Sameshima, Y. and J. Davitz. Suffering as viewed in six different cultures. *American Journal of Nursing* 76 (August 1976), 1296–1297.

Davitz, L. J., Davitz, J. R. and Y. Sameshima. Foreign and American nurses: Reactions and interactions. *Nursing Outlook* 24 (April 1976), 237–242.

Davitz, L. J., Davitz, J. R. and Y. Higuchi. Crosscultural inferences of physical pain and psychological distress, Part I. *Nursing Times* 73 (April 14, 1977), 521–523.

Davitz, L. J., Davitz, J. R. and Y. Higuchi. Crosscultural inferences of physical pain and psychological distress, Part II. *Nursing Times* 73 (April 21, 1977), 556–558.

Davitz, L. J. and J. R. Davitz. Black and white nurses' inferences of suffering. *Nursing Times* 74 (April 27, 1978), 708-710.

Diers, D., Schmidt, L., McBride, B. and L.D. Kette. The effect of nursing interaction on patients in pain. *Nursing Research* 21 (September-October 1972), 419-428.

Graham, L. E. and E. M. Conley. Evaluation of anxiety and fear in adult surgical patients. *Nursing Research* 20 (March-April 1971), 113-122.

Hammond, K. R. Clinical inference in nursing. *Nursing Research* 15 (Summer 1966), 236-243.

Hammond, K. R. Clinical inference in nursing. *Nursing Research* 15 (Fall 1966), 330-336.

Hammond, K. R. Clinical inference in nursing. *Nursing Research* 15 (Winter 1967), 38-45.

Jacox, A. and M. Stewart. *Relation of psychosocial factors and type of pain.* Mimeographed report from the College of Nursing, University of Iowa, Iowa City, 1973.

Johnson, S. B. Relationships between verbal patterns of nursing students and therapeutic effectiveness. *Nursing Research* 13 (Fall 1964), 339-342.

Jourard, S. M. Bedside manner. *American Journal of Nursing* 60 (January 1960), 63-66.

Lenburg, C. B., Davitz, L. J. and H. P. Glass. Inferences of physical pain and psychological distress in relation to the stage of the patient's illness and occupation of the perceiver. *Nursing Research* 19 (September-October 1970), 392-398.

Lester, D., Getty, C. and C. R. Kneisl. Attitudes of nursing students and nursing faculty toward death. *Nursing Research* 23 (January-February 1974), 50-53.

McBride, M. B. Pain and effective nursing practice. *American Nursing Clinical Sessions.* New York: Appleton-Century-Crofts, 1967, 75-82.

McBride, M. B. Nursing approaches, pain, and relief: An exploratory study. *Nursing Research* (Fall 1967), 337-341.

McCaffery, M. and F. Moss. Nursing intervention for bodily pain. *American Journal of Nursing* 67 (June 1967), 1224-1227.

McCaffery, M. *Nursing management of the patient with pain.* Philadelphia: J. B. Lippincott Company, 1972.

Moody, P. M. Attitudes of cynicism and humanitarianism in nursing students and staff nurses. *Journal of Nursing Education* 12 (August 1973), 9-13.

Moss, F. T. and B. Meyer. Effects of nursing interactions upon pain relief in patients. *Nursing Research* 15 (Fall 1966), 303-306.

Newton, M. E., Hunt, W. E., McDowell, W. and A. F. Hanken. *A study of nurse action in relief of pain.* Columbus: The Ohio State University School of Nursing Research Foundation, 1964, 131.

Orlando, A. J. *Dynamic nurse-patient relationship: Function, process and principles.* New York: G. P. Putnam's Sons, 1961.

Petrie, A. *Individuality in pain and suffering.* Chicago: University of Chicago Press, 1967.

Skipper, J. K. and R. C. Leonard. *Social interaction and patient care.* Philadelphia: J. B. Lippincott Company, 1965.

Yeaworth, R. C., Kapp, F. T. and C. Winget. Attitudes of nursing students toward the dying patient. *Nursing Research* 23 (January–February 1974), 20–24.

Zborowski, M. *People in pain.* San Francisco: Jossey Bass, 1969.

Appendix

The Standard Measure of Inferences of Suffering Questionnaire

INSTRUCTIONS

Each of the items in this booklet contains a brief description of a patient. Please read the description of each patient, and then judge the degree of physical pain or discomfort and the degree of psychological stress the patient is probably experiencing. Indicate your judgments about each patient by checking the appropriate places on the two rating scales for each item.

Remember, there are no right or wrong answers. We are only interested in your judgments. Do the ratings as quickly as you can. Don't sit and think for a long time about any one item. Read the description of each patient and quickly size up the case. Then, on the basis of your first reaction to the case, check off the two rating scales, indicating how much physical pain or discomfort and how much psychological distress you feel the patient is experiencing.

		None	Little	Mild	Mod-erate	Great	Severe	VerySevere
1. Tripping on an uneven pavement block, Louise Crane, seventy years of age, fell and sustained a fractured femur. In traction at the moment, surgery is planned.	Physical Pain, Discomfort:	1	2	3	4	5	6	7
	Psychological Distress	1	2	3	4	5	6	7
2. Concerned about the appearance of a mole on her upper left arm, thirty-two year old Elizabeth Burdine decided to have the lesion removed in the doctor's office. The pathology report was negative.	Physical Pain, Discomfort:	1	2	3	4	5	6	7
	Psychological Distress	1	2	3	4	5	6	7
3. Thirty-six year old Gladys Lee stumbled and fell on the sidewalk, sustaining an abrasion of the hand. When the injury was not attended to, an abscess developed which required incision and drainage. She is to care for the hand through soaking and make an appointment to have the hand checked in a few days.	Physical Pain, Discomfort:	1	2	3	4	5	6	7
	Psychological Distress	1	2	3	4	5	6	7
4. Because of a persistent cough and a lingering cold, John Caldwell, age forty, was advised to consult a physician. His condition was diagnosed as broncho-pneumonia requiring hospitalization.	Physical Pain, Discomfort:	1	2	3	4	5	6	7
	Psychological Distress	1	2	3	4	5	6	7
5. While standing on a kitchen chair to reach a high shelf, Nancy Lynch, forty years old, slipped and fractured her right arm. X-rays indicated a fractured radius. The arm was placed in a cast, and now, after six weeks, the cast will be removed.	Physical Pain, Discomfort:	1	2	3	4	5	6	7
	Psychological Distress	1	2	3	4	5	6	7
6. "I expect something to happen to me. I feel I am seeing everything through a new awareness." Forty-one year old Howard Madison reflected his sense of foreboding and feelings of a brighter, clearer world during an intake interview.	Physical Pain, Discomfort:	1	2	3	4	5	6	7
	Psychological Distress	1	2	3	4	5	6	7

		None	Little	Mild	Mod-erate	Great	Severe	Very Severe
7. After a series of tests and examinations, Catherine Kent, forty-two years of age, was hospitalized with thrombophlebitis. Therapeutic measures include anticoagulants and bedrest.	Physical Pain, Discomfort:	1	2	3	4	5	6	7
	Psychological Distress	1	2	3	4	5	6	7
8. Undergoing an annual physical examination, Florence Tully, forty-two years of age was informed that she had a low grade systolic murmur. She has been hospitalized for a series of conclusive tests.	Physical Pain, Discomfort:	1	2	3	4	5	6	7
	Psychological Distress	1	2	3	4	5	6	7
9. Merle Lombard was rushed to the hospital by her mother after this nine year old child fell from a tree-house platform. X-rays indicated a fractured femur, and she has remained at the hospital in traction pending surgery.	Physical Pain, Discomfort:	1	2	3	4	5	6	7
	Psychological Distress	1	2	3	4	5	6	7
10. During a routine psychological test at his school, seven year old Austin Barett appeared troubled and concerned. When asked to arrange a series of blocks according to size and color, he insisted "they have sharp edges," and the "bright colors" bothered him.	Physical Pain, Discomfort:	1	2	3	4	5	6	7
	Psychological Distress	1	2	3	4	5	6	7
11. The general fatigue and behavior of seven year old Madeline Rankin concerned her parents. Seen by a pediatrician, she was admitted to the hospital with a possible diagnosis of leukemia. A complete diagnostic testing program is underway.	Physical Pain, Discomfort:	1	2	3	4	5	6	7
	Psychological Distress	1	2	3	4	5	6	7
12. Concerned about his frequent colds, William Hampton, seventy years old, went to a family doctor. Bronchopneumonia was diagnosed. Mr. Hampton was hospitalized and placed on antibiotic therapy.	Physical Pain, Discomfort:	1	2	3	4	5	6	7
	Psychological Distress	1	2	3	4	5	6	7

		None	Little	Mild	Mod-erate	Great	Severe	Very Severe
13. Concerned about his diffi-culties standing on his feet for any period of time, forty-one year old Martin Downes was examined by his doctor. Thrombophlebitis was diagnosed. Currently he is in the hospital being treated with anticoagulant drugs while on complete bedrest.	Physical Pain, Discomfort:	1	2	3	4	5	6	7
	Psycholog-ical Distress	1	2	3	4	5	6	7
14. While pruning a hedge near his daughter's home, Edward Dennis injured his hand. At the insistence of his daughter, he finally saw a doctor. An incision and drainage of the abscess was performed in the office, and the seventy-two year old man was told to soak his hand and return in three days.	Physical Pain, Discomfort:	1	2	3	4	5	6	7
	Psycholog-ical Distress	1	2	3	4	5	6	7
15. Concerned about a general malaise and an overall feeling of "not being himself," George James, forty years of age, consulted a doctor. Preliminary examination indicated a possi-bility of leukemia, and he is currently hospitalized under-going a diagnostic work-up.	Physical Pain, Discomfort:	1	2	3	4	5	6	7
	Psycholog-ical Distress	1	2	3	4	5	6	7
16. Because of increasing irri-tability over minor concerns and a general feeling of over-sensitivity, Roberta Brower, seventy-two years of age, felt she should seek help from her family physician.	Physical Pain, Discomfort:	1	2	3	4	5	6	7
	Psycholog-ical Distress	1	2	3	4	5	6	7
17. After leaving work, Ray Christopher, sixty-four years old, stumbled on an uneven sidewalk and fractured his femur. Surgery is planned.	Physical Pain, Discomfort:	1	2	3	4	5	6	7
	Psycholog-ical Distress	1	2	3	4	5	6	7

		None	Little	Mild	Mod-erate	Great	Severe	Very Severe
18. Struggling with a toy, five year old Maureen Ferguson hurt her right hand. An abscess developed which the pediatrician incised and drained during an office visit. Maureen's mother was instructed how to soak the child's hand, and to be sure to bring her back to see the doctor in three days.	Physical Pain, Discomfort:	1	2	3	4	5	6	7
	Psychological Distress	1	2	3	4	5	6	7
19. While attempting to change a flat tire on his car, Frank Jordan, thirty-nine years of age, stumbled and struck his arm against the metal jack. The break was set in a cast which remained on the arm for six weeks. He is due to have the cast taken off in a day or so.	Physical Pain, Discomfort:	1	2	3	4	5	6	7
	Psychological Distress	1	2	3	4	5	6	7
20. At the suggestion of a pediatrician, a mole from five year old Joey Herter's right arm was surgically removed in the doctor's office. The pathology report was negative.	Physical Pain, Discomfort:	1	2	3	4	5	6	7
	Psychological Distress	1	2	3	4	5	6	7
21. Observing that Timothy Barnes, a nine year old fourth grader, could not remain seated any length of time and frequently appeared upset by the other children, his teacher sent him to the school nurse. This behavior had occurred with great frequency during the past week.	Physical Pain, Discomfort:	1	2	3	4	5	6	7
	Psychological Distress	1	2	3	4	5	6	7
22. Six year old James Stone was admitted to the hospital. His mother explained that the pediatrician noticed a heart murmur in a routine office examination, and he wanted James to have a complete series of tests.	Physical Pain, Discomfort:	1	2	3	4	5	6	7
	Psychological Distress	1	2	3	4	5	6	7

		None	Little	Mild	Mod-erate	Great	Severe	Very Severe
23. A number of self-concerns about how she was feeling prompted Marcia Claxton, thirty-eight years of age, to check her condition with a doctor. After a preliminary examination and a possible diagnosis of leukemia, hospitalization was deemed necessary for further testing.	Physical Pain, Discomfort:	1	2	3	4	5	6	7
	Psychological Distress	1	2	3	4	5	6	7
24. Eight year old Nancy Sloan had a mole excised from her arm the day before yesterday. She did not require hospitalization, and the biopsy report was negative.	Physical Pain, Discomfort:	1	2	3	4	5	6	7
	Psychological Distress	1	2	3	4	5	6	7
25. Bobby Simpson's mother is bringing him to an orthopedist to have a cast taken off his arm. A month and a half ago, Bobby, a kindergartner, fell from a Jungle Gym in the school playground and sustained a fracture of his right radial bone.	Physical Pain, Discomfort:	1	2	3	4	5	6	7
	Psychological Distress	1	2	3	4	5	6	7
26. Barbara King, forty years of age, told the nurse that many things were disturbing her. She continually worried about the future. Objects appeared to her to be much brighter and clearer than she had ever before experienced.	Physical Pain, Discomfort:	1	2	3	4	5	6	7
	Psychological Distress	1	2	3	4	5	6	7
27. In accordance with his company's requirement, Frederick Britt, age thirty-nine reported for an annual physical examination. The company physician noticed a heart murmur and has requested further tests.	Physical Pain, Discomfort:	1	2	3	4	5	6	7
	Psychological Distress	1	2	3	4	5	6	7
28. Jack Walters, thirty-three, had an excision of a mole from his lower arm done two days ago. The pathology report came back negative.	Physical Pain, Discomfort:	1	2	3	4	5	6	7
	Psychological Distress	1	2	3	4	5	6	7

		None	Little	Mild	Mod-erate	Great	Severe	Very Severe
29. Aware of his growing sense of irritability and general nervous tension at work, George Abbott, forty-four years of age, decided to check out his condition with his personal physician.	Physical Pain, Discomfort:	1	2	3	4	5	6	7
	Psychological Distress	1	2	3	4	5	6	7
30. Stumbling on an icy step, seventy-one year old Charlotte Timmons sustained a fractured left radial bone. Her arm was placed in a cast which has been on for about seven weeks. Her physician has decided that it can now be removed.	Physical Pain, Discomfort:	1	2	3	4	5	6	7
	Psychological Distress	1	2	3	4	5	6	7
31. A series of colds prevented nine year old Lisa Roberts from attending school regularly. As she was unable to get rid of a cough, she was taken to the pediatrician who had the child hospitalized for bronchopneumonia.	Physical Pain, Discomfort:	1	2	3	4	5	6	7
	Psychological Distress	1	2	3	4	5	6	7
32. Marian Benedict injured her hand and the resulting infection concerned her. She went to her doctor who performed an I and D in the office. The seventy-four year old woman is to soak her hand and to return to the physician's office in three days.	Physical Pain, Discomfort:	1	2	3	4	5	6	7
	Psychological Distress	1	2	3	4	5	6	7
33. Seventy-four year old Ernest Trew returned to his doctor's office for a biopsy report on a mole which had been excised from his upper right arm several days previously. The pathology report was negative.	Physical Pain, Discomfort:	1	2	3	4	5	6	7
	Psychological Distress	1	2	3	4	5	6	7
34. Waiting for her turn to be tested, Melanie Stillman, a fourth grader, told the school psychologist that the room light was disturbing. "Everything stands out and bothers me." She complained of feeling "funny" in her stomach.	Physical Pain, Discomfort:	1	2	3	4	5	6	7
	Psychological Distress	1	2	3	4	5	6	7

		None	Little	Mild	Mod-erate	Great	Severe	Very Severe
35. At the insistence of his family doctor, seventy-two year old Henry Marshall has entered the hospital for a complete series of diagnostic studies. An office examination suggested the possibility of leukemia.	Physical Pain, Discomfort:	1	2	3	4	5	6	7
	Psychological Distress	1	2	3	4	5	6	7
36. Retired, Chester Wilcox, age seventy-two, takes the precaution of having annual check-ups. He was notified at his last physical of the presence of a low grade systolic murmur. A diagnostic work-up has been scheduled.	Physical Pain, Discomfort:	1	2	3	4	5	6	7
	Psychological Distress	1	2	3	4	5	6	7
37. Jimmy Falconer, a ten year old boy, caught his finger in a jammed bike gear. An abscess developed which required incision and drainage. The pediatrician told Jimmy's mother how to soak the wound, and instructed her to bring the boy back to see him in a few days.	Physical Pain, Discomfort:	1	2	3	4	5	6	7
	Psychological Distress	1	2	3	4	5	6	7
38. Sixty-six year old Austin Beasly was informed that he had no alternative but to be hospitalized. Diagnosed as having thrombophlebitis, therapy which included bedrest and anticoagulant drugs was begun immediately.	Physical Pain, Discomfort:	1	2	3	4	5	6	7
	Psychological Distress	1	2	3	4	5	6	7
39. "I'm upset, and it's not my usual way," reported Wilma Gray, sixty-seven years of age, to a nurse during an intake interview. She worried, it seemed, about so much. The future, her life--all bothered her. She also said she hadn't changed her glasses, but objects seemed particularly clear to her. "I'm really frightened about the future."	Physical Pain, Discomfort:	1	2	3	4	5	6	7
	Psychological Distress	1	2	3	4	5	6	7

		None	Little	Mild	Mod-erate	Great	Severe	Very Severe
40. Mary Williams, sixty-eight years of age, was notified that a biopsy report was negative. A few days before, her physician had excised a lower arm lesion in an office visit.	Physical Pain, Discomfort:	1	2	3	4	5	6	7
	Psychological Distress	1	2	3	4	5	6	7
41. Jane Patterson, sixty-nine years of age, underwent a routine physical examination prior to obtaining additional insurance. A low grade systolic murmur was noted, and she was told hospitalization was necessary in order for her to have a complete check-up.	Physical Pain, Discomfort:	1	2	3	4	5	6	7
	Psychological Distress	1	2	3	4	5	6	7
42. Lea Hamilton is impatiently waiting for her turn to see the doctor. According to this forty-five year old woman, she has felt high-strung and moody, which she says is not typical of her usual behavior.	Physical Pain, Discomfort:	1	2	3	4	5	6	7
	Psychological Distress	1	2	3	4	5	6	7
43. Fatigue, repeated colds, and a persistent cough prompted thirty-four year old Beth Frawley to seek treatment. Bronchopneumonia was diagnosed and immediate hospitalization required.	Physical Pain, Discomfort:	1	2	3	4	5	6	7
	Psychological Distress	1	2	3	4	5	6	7
44. Complaining of discomfort in her left leg, sixty-seven year old Marie Cunningham made an appointment with her family doctor. The examination indicated thrombophlebitis. Hospitalization was necessary, and she is now being treated with anticoagulant therapy and bedrest.	Physical Pain, Discomfort:	1	2	3	4	5	6	7
	Psychological Distress	1	2	3	4	5	6	7

		None	Little	Mild	Mod-erate	Great	Severe	Very Severe
45. Complaining of general fatigue and malaise, seventy-one year old Rose Walker decided to see her family physician. Examination indicated a need for complete tests to rule out the possibility of leukemia.	Physical Pain, Discomfort:	1	2	3	4	5	6	7
	Psychological Distress	1	2	3	4	5	6	7
46. In traction pending surgery, eleven year old James Foreman sustained a fractured femur when his bike skidded on a wet road and he lost control.	Physical Pain, Discomfort:	1	2	3	4	5	6	7
	Psychological Distress	1	2	3	4	5	6	7
47. Currently on bedrest and receiving anticoagulant therapy, twelve year old William Post was hospitalized with a diagnosis of thrombophlebitis. His parents took him for an examination following the boy's repeated insistence that his "legs hurt."	Physical Pain, Discomfort:	1	2	3	4	5	6	7
	Psychological Distress	1	2	3	4	5	6	7
48. Routinely undergoing an annual physical required by the school, ten year old Jill Cox was found by her pediatrician to have a heart murmur. The physician recommended a thorough hospital examination.	Physical Pain, Discomfort:	1	2	3	4	5	6	7
	Psychological Distress	1	2	3	4	5	6	7
49. Seventy year old Shirly Adams ascribed her continual bouts of colds to the severity of the winter. However, at her family's insistence she did see a doctor who prescribed anti-biotic therapy and insisted she be hospitalized for broncho-pneumonia.	Physical Pain, Discomfort:	1	2	3	4	5	6	7
	Psychological Distress	1	2	3	4	5	6	7
50. Hospitalized and in traction as a result of a fall on an icy street, thirty-nine year old Joan Lawrence has been hospi-talized. Within a few days she'll be having surgery for the fractured femur.	Physical Pain, Discomfort:	1	2	3	4	5	6	7
	Psychological Distress	1	2	3	4	5	6	7

		None	Little	Mild	Mod-erate	Great	Severe	Very Severe
51. Jerome Fleming, thirty-eight years of age, was concerned about the swelling and pain in his hand from an injury he had received at work a week previously. He went to the office clinic and an abscess was incised and drained. After soaking the hand regularly for the next few days, he is due to have the hand checked.	Physical Pain, Discomfort:	1	2	3	4	5	6	7
	Psycholog-ical Distress	1	2	3	4	5	6	7
52. Seventy-three year old Harvey Carpenter customarily followed a routine pattern. Recently, however, he has complained of feeling "edgy" and any suggestion made to him is reacted to with great irritation. The slightest change in schedule makes him nervous.	Physical Pain, Discomfort:	1	2	3	4	5	6	7
	Psycholog-ical Distress	1	2	3	4	5	6	7
53. Concerned about their daughter's complaints of discomfort in her legs, the parents of twelve year old Janet Richards took her for an examination. Throbophlebitis was diagnosed, and Janet entered the hospital to begin treatment which consisted of bedrest and anticoagulants.	Physical Pain, Discomfort:	1	2	3	4	5	6	7
	Psycholog-ical Distress	1	2	3	4	5	6	7
54. Richard Wylie, seventy-two years of age, slipped on an icy pavement six weeks ago. Since that time his fractured arm has been in a cast which his doctor has indicated will be ready to come off in the next day or so.	Physical Pain, Discomfort:	1	2	3	4	5	6	7
	Psycholog-ical Distress	1	2	3	4	5	6	7
55. Noticing Monica Slater's moody and fretful behavior over the last several days, the fifth grade teacher sent the child to see the school nurse.	Physical Pain, Discomfort:	1	2	3	4	5	6	7
	Psycholog-ical Distress	1	2	3	4	5	6	7

		None	Little	Mild	Mod-erate	Great	Severe	Very Severe
56. Benjamin Everett, sixty-five, told the nurse that he'd like an appointment with the doctor as soon as possible. Recently he's been feeling anxious "with waves of anxiety hitting me." He complained of worrying about the future and says he sees everything with great clarity.	Physical Pain, Discomfort:	1	2	3	4	5	6	7
	Psychological Distress	1	2	3	4	5	6	7
57. Six weeks ago, Laurie Jones, a second grader, lost her hold on the school monkey bars and broker her left humerus. An appointment has been made to have the cast removed from the arm.	Physical Pain, Discomfort:	1	2	3	4	5	6	7
	Psychological Distress	1	2	3	4	5	6	7
58. Upon admission to the emergency room following an auto accident, Lewis Knapp, thirty-six years old, was placed immediately in traction. Surgery will be necessary to repair a fractured femur.	Physical Pain, Discomfort:	1	2	3	4	5	6	7
	Psychological Distress	1	2	3	4	5	6	7
59. Eleven year old Stanely Overton seemed unable to shake a cough and cold. Examined by the family physician, his parents were informed that hospitalization and antibiotic therapy were necessary because of broncho-pneumonia.	Physical Pain, Discomfort:	1	2	3	4	5	6	7
	Psychological Distress	1	2	3	4	5	6	7
60. Admitted to the pediatric unit, Peter Goodwin, six years of age, is suspected of having leukemia. At present he is being examined and tested to rule out this possibility.	Physical Pain, Discomfort:	1	2	3	4	5	6	7
	Psychological Distress	1	2	3	4	5	6	7

Index